HOSPICE
A Caring Challenge

By

Elizabeth Gilman McNulty
Chicago, Illinois

and

Robert A. Holderby
Chicago, Illinois

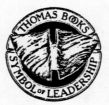

CHARLES C THOMAS • PUBLISHER
Springfield • Illinois • U.S.A.

Published and Distributed Throughout the World by

CHARLES C THOMAS • PUBLISHER
2600 South First Street
Springfield, Illinois, 62717, U.S.A.

© *1983 by* CHARLES C THOMAS • PUBLISHER

ISBN 0-398-04798-7

Library of Congress Catalog Card Number: 82-19245

With THOMAS BOOKS *careful attention is given to all details of
manufacturing and design. It is the Publisher's desire to present books that
are satisfactory as to their physical qualities and artistic possibilities and
appropriate for their particular use.* THOMAS BOOKS *will be true to those
laws of quality that assure a good name and good will.*

Printed in the United States of America

I-R-1

Library of Congress Cataloging in Publication Data

McNulty, Elizabeth G.
    Hospice, a caring challenge.

    Bibliography:p.
    Includes index.
    1. Terminal care.   2. Terminal care facilities.
I. Holderby, Robert A. II. Title. [DNLM: 1. Hos-
pices – United States. 2. Terminal care. WX 28.6 AAl
M4h]
R726.8.M4   1983   362.1'75   82-19245
ISBN 0-398-04798-7

To all of those very special and
remarkable people who care for the terminally ill,
and most especially
to everyone who made a contribution to this book.

67A89

PRACW

PREFACE

". . . PEOPLE can die painlessly, people can die peacefully, and people can die with great dignity.

If hospice can remove the fear of suffering, the fear of being dependent, the fear of being a burden, and the fear of loneliness and isolation, the time will come when death is no longer feared. Death will become what it really is, the natural end of life."

These words of Josefina B. Magno, M. D., former executive director of the National Hospice Organization, reflect the very spirit of the hospice movement in the United States.

This book on the hospice began as an objective, third-person investigation of a concept. It evolved into a first-person experience, which seemed to take on a life of its own because of the remarkable people we encountered along the way.

It was through delving into the history of hospice that we began to understand the unselfish personal involvement of those who have cared for the sick and the dying over the centuries. It was through considering the philosophy of hospice that we renewed our own convictions about quality of life versus quantity of life. It was through a new understanding of the dying person and his needs that our appreciation of hospice grew. It was through our correspondence with pioneer hospice nurses and through our talks with other hospice workers that the circle of our experience became complete.

Our interest in learning about hospice care led us to interviews with those most personally involved . — family members, physicians, nurses, social workers, and volunteers. We looked at hospice through their eyes.

Then we came down to earth to face the practicalities and

problems of hospice care — organizational and financial. We thought seriously about hospice in terms of how it fits into the organization of our health care delivery system and of how it can be — or if it should be — financed in the future.

This book has been a labor of love.

CONTENTS

HOSPICE

Part I
THE CONCEPT

TODAY'S HOSPICE is a way station for sojourners who are making their final journeys. Its philosophy reflects the wholistic concern for easing the physical, emotional, and spiritual pain of the terminally ill person and for sustaining members of his family.

The spreading hospice movement represents a rebirth of the caring concern for persons who are sick and dying — a movement dedicated to helping the patient to live at the same time he is dying. Through acknowledging that recovery is no longer possible for an individual, hospice represents a reversal of commitment to that person. It represents a change of focus from curing to caring.

The hospice story is told here in terms of its basic philosophy, of the people who receive the care, and of the people who give it.

Chapter 1

THE HOSPICE

THROUGHOUT HISTORY, societies and cultures have developed their own "systems of death," which represent the sum total of their beliefs, attitudes, thoughts, feelings, and rituals related to death. From ancient Egypt, where kings were buried with everything they would need in the afterlife, to modern African tribes with their prescribed rites and rituals, peoples have followed their own long-standing traditions related to the final event in a person's life.

In recent history, attitudes toward death and dying have been changing in the Western world, particularly in America. Some 1200 to 1500 years ago, during the Dark Ages, life was viewed as having significance and as being blessed by God. It was imperative, therefore, to maintain the health of the body. This belief was validated by the ceaseless efforts made by doctors in caring for victims of the ravaging epidemics. Later, but prior to the Reformation, the incurably ill in many countries were beloved and prized by the community because the community believed that the Kingdom of Heaven was open to them. The dying were seen as prophets and pilgrims, who gave those around them the opportunity for spiritual growth.

After the Reformation, the sick and dying were no longer considered the holy children of God. Rather, they were believed to be sinners being punished for their evil deeds and ways. This was the attitude in seventeenth and eighteenth century England, where hospitals were simply warehouses for the indigent ill and the criminally insane, who "really deserved no better." (The

5

belief that the ill were being punished for their sins was brought to this country by the Puritans who settled in New England.)

In the nineteenth century, dying and death were recognized as a part of the life cycle, as well as a total family experience. In England, at that time, only the poor died in hospitals. The incurably ill person was cared for by family and physician in his home and he died there.

Since the turn of this century, there has been a gradual shift from this approach, particularly in America, where illness and death have become more and more impersonal. It has been said that death is no longer a subjective, personal experience. It has become an impersonal, objective problem.

With today's modern technology and sophisticated life-support systems, the care of the patient — as well as his fate — has been shifted from the caring environment of the home and the loving ministrations of family members to sterile institutions and to the objective care of impersonal staff members — staff members who are warring against illness and death, not necessarily against pain and suffering.

Since 1900, there has also been an increasing denial of mortality and the reality of death in this country. This denial may be partly the result of Americans' isolation from the reality of death. The dying have been and continue to be ignored. Death has been considered a taboo subject. Moreover, there is considerable evidence that Americans no longer see illness as either the wages of sin or an integral part of the life cycle. Rather, they see it as an infringement on their right to pursue the good life. Since life expectancy has increased over the years, it is easy to consider death as an intrusion, and it is convenient to put off its consideration. These are, perhaps, part of the reason for the slow acceptance of hospice care in this country.

The Hospice Defined

The word *hospice* comes from the Latin word *hospes,* which is the root of such words as hostel, hotel, and hospital. As this root word applies to this alternative approach to patient care, it reflects the meaning of all three.

The basic goal of the modern hospice is to make the patient as comfortable and as clear-headed as possible so that he may function at the highest level he is capable of and enjoy the maximum quality of the life left to him. In general, the hospice seeks to control the patient's pain — emotional and spiritual as well as physical — to help him to have the greatest possible pleasure, to make it possible for him to enjoy social and family relationships, and to help him maintain a positive self-image, so that he may die with dignity.

In order to provide this wholistic concept of care, the hospice focuses on the patient and his family as a single unit. It is the hospice philosophy that the patient should, if at all possible, be in a familiar place surrounded by people and things he loves and that he retain control over his own life as long as he is able.

Interest in wholistic care and family involvement goes back at least to the fourth century before Christ. More than 2,000 years ago, Plato said, "The great error in the treatment of the human body is that physicians are ignorant of the whole." Plato also recommended family involvement and a sympathic approach towards people in extreme personal distress. Albert Schweitzer recognized that patients would be more at ease if they had familiar faces and things around them. Because he recognized this, patients who came to his primitive hospital in French Equatorial Africa in the early part of the twentieth century often brought their entire family with them and most of their animals as well — sheep, goats, chickens, and other miscellaneous animals.

The basic components of hospice care include physican-directed services, control of pain, care by an interdisciplinary team, around-the-clock services, and bereavement services. Whatever the organizational structure, the overriding need is for a comprehensive continuum of care for the patient and the family.

Hospices differ greatly from the American nursing or convalescent homes, which are not usually geared to provide the emotional and spiritual support needed by the patient and his family. Rather, the purpose of the nursing home is to rehabilitate patients so they may return to their communities or to a lower level of care or to provide long-range custodial care when it is not possible or practical for the patient to return to his home or to his community. Hospice care, on the other hand, is characterized by more intensive care by physicians and nurses, by other health care practitioners, and by volunteers. The length of time a person receives hospice care can range from several days to several months, with the average time being about two weeks.

History and Development of the Movement

The modern hospice has a long and rich history, a history that reaches back even beyond the twelfth century, which is often established as the time of the concept's origin. Throughout the centuries, hospice has been a story of loving concern.

Early Hospices

In her book *The Hospice Movement,* Sandol Stoddard presents a fascinating account — through fact and fantasy — of the earliest hospices. She threads a giant tapestry with rich pictures of European and Middle Eastern hospices, tracing their origins back to several hundred years after the birth of Christ. Two of the earliest known hospices, she tells us, were the hospice at Turmanin in Syria, dating back to 475 A.D., and one founded sometime earlier in Rome to care for the pilgrims coming back from Africa.

In Medieval times and earlier, hospices were havens providing shelter and caring concern for pilgrims and wayfarers on their way to the Holy Land, for crusaders going to take the Holy Land from the Moslems, and for children and the indigent. These early hospices, many of them founded by religious orders, flourished in England and in Europe. In Medieval England, even though the population was small, there were reported to be 750 hospices. At that time, there were about 40 in Paris and 30 in Florence.

The following mandate of a twelfth century hospital in England reflects the caring spirit of the hospice.

> If anyone in infirm health and destitute of friends should seek admission for a term until he shall recover, let him be gladly received and assigned a bed. In regard to the poor people who are received late at night, to go forth early in the morning, let the warden take care that their feet are washed and, as far as pos-

sible their necessities attended to.[1]

As the Middle Ages came to a close in the fifteenth century, hospices as places of shelter and caring began receding from the pages of history. In sixteenth century England, where hospices once thrived, monasteries were being closed and nursing orders were being dispersed. Property was being redistributed among already wealthy landowners.

Although many hospices were fading into obscurity, the spirit remained. It lived on in such places as the Gheel community in Belgium, which has provided "foster care" since those Medieval times. It lived on in the hospice for galley slaves founded by the priest Vincent de Paul in seventeenth century France. He had, himself, been sold into slavery after being captured by pirates. Vincent de Paul also founded a nursing order called the Sisters of Charity. The spirit of hospice lived on in eighteenth century Germany where a Protestant minister founded Kaiswerwerth, the first Protestant hospital to have an order of nursing sisters or deaconesses. Kaiserwerth was devoted to caring for the destitute sick and dying.

Spread of the Movement

In the eighteenth and nineteenth centuries, the hospice movement began to thrive once more. Its history includes such names as Elizabeth Fry, who worked for hospital and prison reform in England, and Florence Nightingale, the Lady with the Lamp. It was a one-time co-worker of Florence Nightingale, Sister Mary Aikenhead, who was responsible for the rebirth of the hospice movement in Great Britain. Through her inspiration, the Irish Sisters of Charity founded Our Lady's Hospice at Harold's Cross just outside of Dublin in 1879. Sister Mary Aikenhead did not live to see her dream come true; she died in 1858.

Interestingly, the May 1835 issue of the *Dublin Penny Journal* gave this description of the area in which the Sisters of Charity founded their hospice:

---

[1] DuBois, Paul M. *The Hospice Way of Death.* (New York: Human Sciences Press, 1980.)

> Scarcely one mile from the castle, in the direction of the Grand
> Canal, is a pleasant village. The air in this neighborhood has long
> been considered particularly favourable to invalids; and the vil-
> lage has therefore been much frequented by persons in a delicate
> state of heath.[2]

Another of the early hospices was founded halfway around the
world in Australia. It is the Sacred Heart Hospice, founded by the
Sisters of Charity in 1890.[3] Still another early hospice — one that
foreshadowed the dynamics of the twentieth century hospice —
was founded in London before the turn of the century. It was St.
Luke's Home, founded by Dr. Howard Barrett in 1893. Yet another early hospice was St. Joseph's, which was founded — also in
London — in 1905.

It was not until 1958, however, when Dame Cicely Saunders
began her work at St. Joseph's, that the modern hospice movement began to gain momentum. As a result of her work there,
and with an initial gift of 500 pounds from a dying patient, she
was able, in 1967, to establish St. Christopher's Hospice in Syden-
ham just outside of London.

Inevitably, the rekindling of the hospice spirit radiated out
from Great Britain. It crossed the Atlantic Ocean to the United
States and Canada and crossed the English Channel to Europe
and the Middle East and on to the Far East.

Hospice in America

A few not-for-profit institutions had been founded in America
prior to the turn of the century, for the purpose of caring for
dying patients — dying patients who were indigent. Among them
were Calvary Hospital in New York City and Youville Hospital
in Cambridge, Massachusetts.

However, it was a later combination of events that gave the real
impetus to the hospice movement in this country — a visit to
Yale University by Dame Cicely Saunders, the work of Elisabeth Kubler-Ross, Carl Nighswonger, and others who began study-

---

[2] Butler, Sister Katherine. *We Help Them Home.* (Dublin: Our Lady's Hospice, 1979.)
[3] Personal Correspondence with Sr. Mary Patricia O'Donnell, Sacred Heart Hospice,
August 4, 1982.

ing and writing about death and dying, and a growing national dissatisfaction with the care being given to patients who were terminally ill.

When Dame Cicely lectured at Yale in 1963, her audience included Florence Wald of the University's Graduate School of Nursing. Florence Wald was to play an important part in the growth of the hospice movement in the United States, becoming a pioneer in the movement and one of the founders of the free-standing Connecticut Hospice, in Cambridge, Massachusetts, one of the earliest such organizations in the United States.

Opening the door to acceptance of the hospice concept in this country were the early studies of the subject of death. Prior to the 1959 publication of *The Meaning of Death,* a series of essays edited by Henry Fiefel, very little serious study had been given to the subject. However, the publication, in 1970, of *On Death and Dying* by Elisabeth Kubler-Ross is credited with being the catalyst to the acceptance and development of hospice care in this country.

The growing dissatisfaction with the care being given to terminally ill patients had its roots in modern technology and in the prevailing attitude toward the dying person. The high technology that has invaded, and all but taken over, medical care in recent years has, too often, made that care impersonal and dehumanizing. Machines are taking over the care of the patient, simply to maintain life.

Because of attitudes toward dying persons, particularly in acute-care hospitals, many patients spend their last days in terrifying and lonely isolation. Many physicians and nurses, trained to save lives with high technology care, consider the dying patient to be a failure and often avoid him. Many times, the patient also comes to see himself in that light.

Until recently, medical and nursing education programs did not include courses on death and dying or on relating to the terminally ill patient and his family. The resulting inability to cope has often led practitioners to avoid the dying patient when possible. Yet, dying like birthing requires some help. Now, universities, teaching hospitals, theological seminaries, and nursing schools are offering courses on death and dying.

Avoiding the dying person is not limited to medical and health care practitioners. A 1966 study by Richard Kalish[4] showed that people were more likely to avoid the dying person than they were to avoid members of some of the minority and ethnic groups that are often discriminated against — even if the dying person were a friend or neighbor.

Hospices around the World

Spreading into Europe and beyond, the hospice movement has taken on different characteristics as the result of population, demographics, and social and political systems in these countries. In many countries in Europe, the hospice concept is reflected not so much in hospice institutions and programs as it is in education of health care and social work professionals in the theory and techniques of palliative care — care that is designed to alleviate pain and suffering, rather than to cure or rehabilitate. In the Scandinavian countries, for example, there are no hospices, because all health care practitioners in Norway, Sweden, and Denmark are trained in palliative care.[5]

On the other hand, just across the North Sea in the Netherlands, a great deal of interest is being shown in the hospice movement. While nursing and convalescent homes in the Netherlands have, for many years, treated, nursed, and counseled patients who were terminally ill, they are expanding their efforts in this area. A foundation called Beyond the Last City has been founded for, among other reasons, establishing centers for counseling and caring for the terminally ill.[6]

There has also been some interest in hospice care in the Middle East where, in the fall of 1981, the Israeli Ministry of Health authorized his country's first hospice in Tel Aviv.[7] Further east, hospices are flourishing in Japan and in the Philippines. The

---

[4] Kalish, Richard A. Social distance and the dying. *Community Mental Health Journal* 2(2):152 February-March 1966.
[5] Swedish Ministry of Health and Social Affairs. *I livets slutskede* (Stockholm: The Ministry, 1979), and personal correspondence with Fanny Hartmann (Denmark), April 28, 1982.
[6] Personal correspondence with F.J.G. Oostvogel, M.D., University of Leiden, April 27, 1982.
[7] Personal correspondence with E. Robinson, M.D., October 12, 1981.

movement is growing, too, in Austrialia, with hospices located in Kell and in Brisbane, as well as the Sacred Heart Hospice in Darlinghurst.

State of the Art in America

While hospices in the United States are similar in many ways to those in Great Britain, there are subtle differences between them in organization, structure, and style that relate to culture and tradition and to our political, social, and economic systems, as well as to our health care delivery system.

In Great Britain, the center of the hospice movement has been the freestanding, autonomous institution, providing comprehensive home-care services as well as inpatient care. Most of the institutions also provide hospital back-up. Some patients can be cared for mainly in the home, but come to the hospice for reevaluation or pain control measures or for giving respite to the family.

In the United States, only a small percentage of care is provided in freestanding institutions. The greatest percentage, almost 50 percent, is provided by hospital-based programs, some with inpatient beds, and the rest by community-based programs. Some hospitals having inpatient beds have special units or wings; in other hospitals, hospice patients are cared for throughout the institution. The most recent entry into the hospice field is the nursing home. Although not widespread as yet, some nursing homes are adding hospice units or wings to their facilities.

Whatever the organizational basis, the hospice care is provided by a physician-directed team that almost invariably includes a nurse, a social worker, a pastoral counselor, a dietician, and volunteers who help with the various activities of daily living. Sometimes these services are provided by consultants, other times they are provided by actual members of the team.

Despite the perceived need for a more human and sensitive approach to patient care in this country, hospice care has met with a number of obstacles — financial, organizational, legal and ethical, and psychological. Two major obstacles — the financial and organizational obstacles — are discussed briefly here and then in more detail in Part III of this book.

Funding is one of the major problems facing hospices today.

Although costs can be dramatically reduced if care is given in the home, insurers have been slow to provide for hospice care in their contracts. A 1981 survey of a representative sample of third-party payors showed little support for hospice care.[8] The study indicated that the lack of support was caused, in part, by a general confusion about hospice as an alternative form of care. It was also caused by concern over the fact that no principles or standards had been developed for governing and guiding the future development of hospice services.

Recently, however, some insurance carriers, such as Blue Cross/ Blue Shield, have been experimenting with pilot programs incorporating hospice care. In the fall of 1981, Representative Leon Panetta, of California, introduced a bill in the U.S. Congress for the extension of Medicare benefits to cover hospice services.[9] While, in general, hope has been expressed for the passage of the measure, some people see it as a mixed blessing. There are those who believe that if the federal government includes hospice coverage in Medicare that Blue Cross/Blue Shield and the commercial carriers will not be far behind in covering it. There are other people who worry that Medicare coverage will open the door for profit-hungry entrepreneurs who will care less about the patients and families than they will about the size of their profits. Still others are concerned that, since hospice is less costly than in-patient care, cost reduction not good palliation will become the national priority for hospice.

In addition to the problem of covering the cost of services, there is the problem of funding for the development of hospice programs. Funding has had to come, as available, from private foundations, community resources, private contributions, etc.

Almost as important as the financial problem is the organizational problem of integrating the hospice into the existing system — a system caught up in inertia and one that is slow to accept radical change. Hospitals and other health care facilities are organized for providing sophisticated curative care. Fitting the hospice into the complex delivery system is further compounded

---

[8] Hospice Reimbursement Study, conducted by Frank B. Hall Consulting Company, October 1981.
[9] The bill was passed by the 97th Congress on August 19, 1982.

by the several hospice models and several different types of organizations and institutions providing the care, each with its own possibilities and problems.

There are also legal and ethical obstacles to the rapid spread of the hospice concept in this country. These include federal regulations related to health care facilities, state licensure and other state regulations, standards and principles, to say nothing of the accreditation of programs and national public policy related to the allocation of scarce resources. Legislation affecting hospitals, nursing homes, and home health agencies does not yet apply to hospice programs. Only two states have established licensing requirements for hospice programs. The Joint Commission on Accreditation of Hospitals, basically an institution-oriented organization, is in the process of developing standards for hospice care.

Included among other problems are the time and experience needed to develop standards and principles and the time and experience required to develop education programs and materials and to train the generations of practitioners and volunteers needed to make the hospice concept viable.

Future of the Movement

If the hospice movement grows and gains momentum in this country, care will be most likely provided in the patient's home. Many persons now involved in hospice care believe the most viable model will be the hospital-based home-care program or the program that is closely affiliated with a hospital.

The major, but by no means the only, factor that will affect the growth of the hospice movement here will be financing — sources, methods, and adequacy. Early funding provided through federal funding of demonstration projects, private and community contributions, foundation grants, and so forth will have to be replaced by ongoing and permanent sources of financing.

If adequate funding is not available, only those hospices with substantial private funding or with the resources of a hospital behind them are likely to survive over the long term. Even with a great percentage of care being provided by volunteers (professional and nonprofessional), hospice care can be costly to the program and to the patient — although not nearly as costly as acute care in the hospital.

Other vitally important factors that will shape hospices in the future will be acceptance of the basic philosophy by the medical community at large and a new focus on palliative care in medical and nursing education programs in this country.

Community understanding and acceptance of the concept is another factor that will be reflected in the demand for hospice services. To date, there has been no groundswell of support for the concept. If the concept does become widely accepted, however, original demands for services may be misleading and may result in unrealistic expansions of programs or services. Most hospice care is home care. Because of the toll that such care takes on members of the family, many family members find they are unable — physically, psychologically, or emotionally — to care for their loved one, no matter how much they may want to do it. For this reason, many people believe that a relatively small number of hospices will be able to meet the demand for hospice care.

Akin to the problem of whether family members will be able to care for the dying loved one is the concern that there may not be enough people, both professional and nonprofessional, who will be able to deal with death and dying on a regular basis over long periods of time. It is the belief of many that burnout will be a serious problem for hospice caregivers.

In the best of all possible worlds, however, proponents see hospice care becoming an integral part of the continuum of health care delivery — one that is fully covered by health insurance, whether care is provided in the home or in an institution. As hospice is brought into the mainstream of health care delivery, they see a corresponding change being made in medical and nursing education programs, which will incorporate courses in death and dying, palliative care, and human relations skills for all future physicians and nurses.

This change in the system will begin to happen when physicians can comfortably say, "I can no longer cure you, but I can go on caring for you."

Chapter 2

HOSPICE: Reversal of Commitment

THE sprawling building complex is an internationally known medical center — a place where miracles occur almost daily. Within its walls are found the most advanced specialty units, services, and programs, from nuclear medicine to hospice care. It is also a hub of medical research, where white-coated scientists in ultramodern laboratories are waging war against illness and death.

People come to this center from the four corners of the earth to be treated by its nationally and internationally known physicians, physicians who are supported by highly trained professionals from every specialty and subspecialty and by the most sophisticated diagnostic and therapeutic equipment available.

In waging his all-out battle against death, the physician in this medical center has at his disposal a CT scanner, a cobalt unit, hemocult screening equipment, a digital imager, echocardiograph equipment, mobile gamma cameras, computerized medical records, etc.

On the second floor of the most modern building is the oncology unit. There is a sudden flurry of activity in room 203 — the room of Anita Fleming, a terminally ill cancer patient. Mrs. Fleming has just returned from the first in her second series of cobalt treatments. Her moans are audible over the hustle and bustle of the activity of getting her settled back in bed. When the nurses have made the patient as comfortable as possible, they move on to the next patient who needs them. Mrs. Fleming's room once again becomes quiet and lonely and ominous, and she has time to wonder why the doctors and nurses seldom come

17

to see her anymore.

During these past few months of her illness, Anita Fleming has been cared for by a top-flight medical team — one that includes her internist, an oncologist, oncology nurses, highly specialized and highly trained laboratory technologists, etc.

The team has tried every technique and procedure at its disposal to prolong her life. They give her medication whenever the pain becomes unbearable. Mrs. Fleming's physicians and nurses have refused to acknowledge and share with her the fact of her imminent death. How do they know that she needs time to make arrangements for her elderly and mentally impaired mother, who will be totally alone when Mrs. Fleming dies? What do they know and understand of the patient's fear and isolation as she lives out the last few moments of her life in that sterile and forboding room?

On the floor above is another specialty unit — the hospice unit — where another patient, Elmer Swanson, is terminally ill with cancer. His bright, flower-filled room looks nothing like its counterparts in other areas of the hospital. It is not a maze of machines and equipment, tubes, and intravenous feeding stands.

A young woman — a volunteer — is sitting beside Mr. Swanson's bed. A close look will show that she is holding his hand. The two are engrossed in earnest conversation about the kind of "no frills" funeral he wants to have. The conversation is punctuated with gentle laughter.

Almost unnoticed, a nurse slips into the room to give Mr. Swanson a routine injection for controlling his pain. The patient's medication schedule has been carefully monitored by the physician member of the hospice team, and injections are given before the pain has a chance to begin. Through the regular monitoring of the medication, the physician has found that the medication's buildup now makes it possible to reduce the dosage with no adverse effect on his patient.

A photograph of Mr. Swanson's family stands prominently on the bedside table, and there are other homey touches in the pleasant room. The only indication of the seriousness of Mr. Swanson's illness is the oxygen outlet over the head of his bed.

Soon, the photograph seems to come to life, as family members spill into the room — even his young grandson is permitted to visit him. Mr. Swanson's face lights up as he gives his grandson a wink and a warm smile. Family members are here to visit grandpa, but they are also here to feed him and to get him settled for the night. The family hopes that it will soon be possible to take care of grandpa at home, with the help of the hospital's hospice team. He had come to the hospital for symptom and pain control measures.

Mr. Swanson's room is filled with warmth and joy and laughter. After dinner and a game of chess with his grandson — his daughter helps him move the pieces — the family prepares to go home. Mr. Swanson's daughter helps him into the bathroom and then back into bed. She puts his denture into a container on the bedside table and makes sure that the call bell is within reach. Then the family members step out into the quiet corridor. As they walk down the hall, they pass a comfortably furnished lounge where patients are talking with members of their families. In the small kitchen off the lounge, a group of patients are having coffee and cake. There is no bustle here.

Because the professionals who are caring for Mr. Swanson have been open and honest with him and his family, the patient has been able to make some important decisions, to "set his house in order." The members of the family, with the support of the hospice team, have been able to deal with the loss to come and to begin the healthy process of letting go, of withdrawing the investment of intense feelings they have for Mr. Swanson.

One of the decisions Mr. Swanson has made is to go home to die. Mr. Swanson does go home. He enjoys the last few weeks of his life, virtually pain free, surrounded by his beloved family. He is sitting on the patio overlooking his flower-filled garden, on a beautiful spring morning, when he dies — a contented and peaceful smile on his face. Two of his cats rest comfortably on his feet.

Hospice care represents a nearly total reversal of the practitioner's basic commitment to the patient. In America, particularly, physicians and nurses are committed to prolonging life at almost any cost. They are trained to use everything at their command, from sophisticated technology to advanced medication therapy, to keep the patient alive — no matter what the quality of that life is. To many practitioners, impending death represents failure. Because health care personnel usually experience so much anxiety in caring for the dying patient, they often take refuge in doing the routine, technical, and impersonal tasks involved in patient care, in order to keep from developing a personal relationship with that patient. Often physicians and nurses avoid the dying patient if at all possible.

Ben Yeager was a big, robust, outgoing construction worker — a person that everyone liked. When he went into the hospital he made friends, immediately, with all the doctors, nurses, aides, and maintenance people. Although he did not know it, he had a rapidly growing form of cancer.

The patient began to deteriorate rapidly. The more he deteriorated, the fewer visits he had from his hospital friends. It puzzled and hurt him that the people who used to stick their heads in his room so often weren't coming to see him anymore. So Ben Yeager made feeble jokes about having body odor.

In hospice care, nurses, social workers, and other members of the team are committed to enhancing the quality of the patient's life, not to extending the quantity of life. Hospice care focuses on low technology not high technology, on caring not curing, and on caring for the family not just caring for the patient alone. Hospice care combines sophisticated pain and symptom control procedures with attention and tender loving care.

Low Technology Care

Low technology hospice care relies heavily on sophisticated pain control methods designed to keep the patient clearheaded as well as comfortable and functional. It also relies on the continuing evaluation of the medication — dosage, effectiveness, and side effects — with changes made as needed. Unlike many of their counterparts in acute-care medicine, most hospice practitioners believe in controlling pain before it begins. As has been said,

"You don't wait for a diabetic coma before giving a patient insulin, do you?"

The advanced pain control medications now available do not change the patient's personality or alter or impair his alertness. Instead, they make it possible for him to make the best use of the time he has left, to function at the highest level possible, to do things he needs to do (as in the case of Mrs. Fleming), and to say his goodbyes. These medications and the loving care that goes with them make it possible for the patient to live until he dies.

Some of the most effective pain control medications are not yet permitted in this country because they include the use of controlled substances, most notably heroin. In England, for example, an early medication called the Brompton cocktail was a mixture that included heroin, cocaine, ethyl alcohol, syrup, and chloroform water. Although Great Britain and more than thirty-five other countries permit the closely supervised medical use of heroin, the United States has, until recently, been adamant in its stand against the legal use of the drug. Some would argue the possibility of drug addiction among terminally ill patients. However, would addiction be all that bad in the final days or weeks of their lives?

In March of 1982, a ray of hope appeared. Daniel Inouye, a senator from Hawaii, introduced a bill in the United States Congress that would permit the very carefully controlled use of heroin in the care of terminally ill patients.

"I'm fighting a losing battle with bone cancer," one person wrote in support of the legislation. "I'm now 72, lived a full life, and ask no sympathy, but I would like a chance to compete with the street junkies for a substance that could lessen my problems." Another wrote, "My wife has been fighting cancer for ten years. . . She's now in the terminal stage, and all the medication the doctors have tried do no good. She gets 600 milligrams a day of morphine — for one or two hours of relief."[1]

Although heroin mixtures have been found to be very effective in controlling pain, there are other mixtures of oral medications that are effectively being used in this country.

Pain control is not the whole story. Often, the patient has

---

[1] Excerpts from letters received by the National Committee on the Treatment of Intractible Pain.

severe discomfort — symptoms of the disease or side effects of medication being given — such as nausea, vomiting, and drowsiness. Despite the effectiveness of the drugs now being used for pain and symptom control, research continues in this area.

Caring not Curing

With its emphasis on caring not curing, the hospice offers a high staff/volunteer to patient ratio. Only in this way can it truly provide for the medical, emotional, and spiritual needs of the patient and for the emotional and bereavement services for the family — services that are available around-the-clock.

Whether the patient is being cared for at home, in an acute-care hospital, in a nursing home that provides hospice care, or in a free-standing hospice, the care is based on an evaluation of the patient and his needs and on an evaluation of the emotional and psychological strength of members of his family. If the patient is to be cared for at home, an evaluation is also made of the physical and emotional ability of family members to care for the patient and of the physical environment in the home.

The physician member of the hospice team is responsible for continued monitoring of pain and symptom control measures, altering them as necessary, to maintain an effective level of functioning and relating to family members and friends. Other professional members of the team help with the physical and emotional care of the patient, according to his particular needs. Sometimes, but not always, skilled nursing care is needed. Sometimes the patient needs the skills of a physical therapist, a speech therapist, a pastoral counselor, or a nutritionist. These professionals may actually be members of the team or they may provide consulting services to it.

All members of the team are involved in sharing information and teaching basic skills to members of the patient's family. This may include instructing the patient's husband in how to prepare her food in the blender to make it possible for the patient to eat instead of being fed intravenously.

Perhaps the caring approach is most visibly reflected in the time and attention given by volunteers. Because of the "high person, low technology" care given, most hospices rely heavily on volunteers. Without volunteers the cost of such care would be prohibitive. A look at a cross section of volunteers would, in all probability, show an interesting mix — health care professionals doing such nonprofessional work as chauffeuring small children to nursery school and persons from other walks of life shopping for groceries or negotiating for a hospital bed.

People seem to be very drawn to the hospice idea, and they are very special kinds of people. Volunteers are drawn to hospice care for many reasons. Some simply want to help, others want to give of themselves because of an experience good or bad they have had in their own lives, still others have had friends or relatives who have been cared for by hospice programs. Sometimes retired people volunteer to help fill up their days or because in retirement they have time to give. Some people feel the need to come to terms with their own deaths or, perhaps, to prepare for the loss of a loved one.

Volunteers perform a variety of services — services that depend on the specific needs of the patient and his family, on the volunteer's own particular skills, on the makeup of the team, and on program and community resources.

Patient/Family Unit

Unlike most acute-care professionals, hospice personnel consider the patient and his family the "unit" of care. It has been said that ignoring the family of the dying patient is to ignore the very framework of the patient's existence. It is also to deny the wholistic approach to patient care, because caring for the "whole patient" means caring for the family too. In some cases, the family needs more care and attention than the patient does.

Because persons closest to the dying patient usually constitute a natural support system, use of this spontaneous human asset is vital and invaluable. Helping family members strengthen that support system helps remove the barrier between the dying patient and members of his family.

Members of the hospice team help both the patient and the family members come to terms with the impending death. Coming to terms often breaks down the communications barrier between them, so that the patient is not alone, mentally or emotionally —

made that way because those nearest to him cannot bear to share the anguish of his last moments.

In most cases, the patient needs to talk openly and honestly about his death, about how he feels about dying, and about plans or arrangements he needs to make. He needs to begin his leave taking and get ready to say his goodbyes, as do those who love him. He may need to resolve conflicts in family relationships. These things can only be done when everyone involved is able to come to terms with the death and is able to speak about it.

A minister, who has counseled many dying patients and their families, usually can get family communication going by simply saying to the patient, "Tell me about your illness." As often as not, the patient responds with some variation of "I've got cancer and I am dying." Once it is out in the open, the barriers begin to come down and the patient and family begin to take the first steps toward exploring and understanding their own and each other's feelings.

The need for coming to terms is often overlooked in acute-care medicine, where physicians often do not tell the patient he is dying and forbid members of the staff to discuss it. Some physicians refuse to discuss the patient's prognosis with members of the family. When the physician withholds all information, tension often begins to grow between the questioning family members and the always uninformative staff. The tension then may become friction, and if the friction increases unchecked, the care of the patient may deteriorate.

Fortunately, attitudes are changing and health care practitioners are recognizing the importance of openness and honesty with the patient and his family. Failure to help them in this way can have long-range repercussions. These repercussions are reflected in the plight of the widow and children of a man who had no will and whose finances were in chaos or in the tragic situation of the young widower who almost lost his fledgling business because he was totally unprepared to be both mother and father to his five small children.

It is generally believed that persons closest to the patient should be encouraged to take part in the day-to-day care of the patient, as a way of experiencing the death and as a way of receiving emotional support. Sometimes members of the family want to provide all of the care. Not everyone can do that, however — either for emotional or physical reasons. For those who can provide all or most of the care, the experience can be emotionally satisfying and rewarding.

In one of the dialogues in Part II of this book, a young woman talks about her emotional need to help care for her mother and about her pride in being able to do such things as change oxygen tanks, keep a record of her mother's medication, and insert a catheter. It was extremely important for that daughter and for other members of her family to work with the hospice team in caring for their beloved mother.

Members of the hospice team make it possible for people like Cindy Mitchell to fill the need to help with the physical care of the loved one. They do this by sharing information and teaching basic skills. Many times members of the hospice team help family members by explaining how the disease will progress and what the family should expect at the time of the patient's death. Skill teaching may include such things as how to give a massage, how and how often to move the patient to prevent bed sores, how to get the patient out of bed and into a chair, or how to monitor the oxygen supply.

Hospice caregivers also provide information, emotional and spiritual support, and counseling during the patient's illness and after the patient's death. Those close to the dying person are encouraged to continue to live their own lives during the dying process. They are encouraged to continue to maintain the continuity of their normal lives and their outside activities. Doing so makes it easier for family members to pick up the pieces and return to a normal life after the patient's death. It often makes it easier for the patient, too, who may worry about being a burden or about drastically changing his loved one's lives if their own lives are centered on him.

When death comes over a protracted period of time, as it usually does with hospice patients, loved ones have an opportunity to begin the process of letting go. During the mutual and healthy withdrawal of invested feelings, family members need to explore and understand their individual responses to what is going on and how they feel about what is going on and, in fact, how they feel toward the dying person. They also have to learn how to deal with all of these feelings.

Sometimes the simple sharing of thoughts and feelings over the course of time is all the support the individual needs. Other times family members need to be assured that some seemingly outrageous feelings they may be having — anger, rejection, self-pity, hate — are acceptable feelings and, in many cases, appropriate and expected. They need help in recognizing, accepting, and dealing with the love-hate relationship they may be having with the dying person. Sometimes family members need more than simple sharing and listening. The effective hospice team, alert to the possibility and sensitive to individual needs, may recommend and/or provide psychological or psychiatric counseling.

With many hospices, bereavement service means more than simply supporting the family in the days immediately following the death and through the funeral. It may mean as long as a year's follow-up to be sure that members of the family have gone through the natural grief process, have come out the other side, and are living well adjusted and productive lives.

The reversal of commitment in the hospice philosophy reflects the growing awareness of the need and the right of each individual to live — really live — while he dies and to die with dignity, surrounded by love and affection.

Chapter 3

THE HOSPICE PATIENT

HOSPICE patients, by definition, have a single bond in common — a limited life span. While, today, most persons receiving hospice care are cancer patients, terminality is the single common denominator.

Most dying patients go through the five stages in the acceptance of death described in 1970 by Elisabeth Kubler-Ross. They also share many of the same feelings of anger, fear, rejection, anxiety, isolation, and many other emotions as they face the ultimate experience of life.

Most, if not all, hospices require that the patient and his family know and understand both the diagnosis and the prognosis of the patient's condition, whether they choose to deny them or not. Because a patient may be admitted to a hospice program anytime from several months to several days after learning of his prognosis, he may be at any stage in the final acceptance of his terminality.

Although much has been written about the five stages of accepting impending death — denial and isolation, anger, bargaining, depression, and final acceptance — they are reviewed here, briefly, in terms of the patient and his family. While these are identifiable stages, they may not come in the order given here, they may blur together, or one or more stages may be repeated, and repeated more than one time. One patient, for example, may have reached the stage of depression and then reverted to the denial stage. Another patient may not go through the denial stage first. He may begin with anger.

Stages in Acceptance

Often the patient's first response to being told he has a ter-

27

minal illness is one of disbelief. "It can't be! This happens to other people! Not me!" Many times this disbelief and denial lead to isolation — emotional and sometimes physical. Isolating himself may, perhaps, be the patient's way of avoiding the reality. By not letting family members and friends get close to him, the patient may, for a while, be able to continue his denial.

Usually, the second stage is anger. In asking why this terrible thing has happenened to him, the patient goes over all of the reasons why it shouldn't be happening to him, and his anger often increases. If the patient is religious, his anger may be turned toward his God. If he is not, it may be directed at the "incompetence" of his physician, or it may even be directed at family members or friends. It is an emotion that must be expressed.

When the patient is in the angry stage, he is often difficult to care for and even to deal with on any level. He may express his anger openly and often — refusing to cooperate with caregivers or family members. He may become verbally abusive to those around him or he may refuse to even talk to them. Sometimes the patient's personality appears to undergo a change — temporary or permanent. The ordinarily mild-mannered, wellspoken person may resort to outbursts of verbal obscenities and cutting, sarcastic remarks.

The patient's anger often poses a threat to the persons caring for him, whether those persons are health care professionals or whether they are members of his family. Expressed anger can also engender negative thoughts in those persons — conflicting, angry, guilty thoughts — which will affect the patient, his care, and those around him.

In the bargaining stage, the patient will bargain with his doctor, or with his God, or with himself. He will bargain in any way that he thinks will work the miracle he needs. If he is bargaining with his doctor, he will promise any and every kind of cooperation and every effort to eliminate self-destructive actions or overindulgences. If he is bargaining with his God, he will return to his religion with fervor and promise to lead an exemplary life from here on in; he may remind his God of his faithfulness and good works, promising to do even better in the future.

Sometimes the patient is simply bargaining for a brief postponement of the inevitable — a postponement for the woman who wants to live to see the birth of her first grandchild, a postponement for the father who wants to see his son graduate from law school, a postponement for the mother who wants to attend her daughter's wedding, a postponement for the person who wants to get his house in order and make arrangements for his family.

In the depression stage, the patient often turns all of his anger and his frustration inward. This is what Kubler-Ross calls reactive depression. In this state of depression, the patient may be irritable and troublesome or he may become remote and uncommunicative. Reactive depression is most often triggered by self-anger. The anger may be caused by feelings of guilt or shame for things done or for things not done, or it may be caused by the angry feeling that fate has played a cruel joke on him. Whatever the cause, reactive depression is an angry reaction in which the anger is turned inward.

Kubler-Ross identifies another type of depression — anticipatory or preparatory depression. Preparatory depression is not triggered by anger. Rather, it is caused by the anticipation of the loss that the impending death will bring — the loss of loved ones and love objects. Preparatory depression is one of the ways a dying patient begins to let go. It usually comes just before final acceptance.

Final acceptance is usually reflected in calmness and serenity and in a willingness to let go. Experience of pastoral counselors and crisis intervention counselors has shown that the majority of people — at the moment of death — accept death in peace and tranquility.

The patient had come into the hospital with an exceedingly fast-growing skin cancer. One night, after being in the hospital for about a week, he asked the chaplain to come in to see him. They talked for three hours about the patient's feelings — his anger, frustration, and bitterness and also about his joys and his happiness. The Chaplain listened quietly. When he got the sign to leave, the chaplain got up and bid the patient goodnight.

The next day, the chaplain came by to see the patient once more. When he asked the patient if he wanted to talk, the patient responded, "No, I'm all talked out. I've resolved my conflicts. The time has come." Within three hours, the patient had died a peaceful and serene death.

There is evidence now that the dying person's loved ones go through those same five stages in much the same way as the patient does. Often, however, it is a matter of delayed reaction, with the loved ones coming to each stage after the patient does. Whenever it happens, the needs and reactions are similar.

Special Feelings, Concerns, and Needs

For most persons, illness and/or hospitalization brings on feelings of fear and anxiety, feelings of separation and isolation, and feelings of helplessness and dependence. While the feelings, concerns, and needs of the dying patient are similar to those of most other patients, there are some striking differences — some very special concerns and needs.

Almost all patients have feelings of fear and anxiety when faced with illness, particularly serious illness. They fear the diagnosis. They fear the prognosis. They fear bodily mutilation as a result of surgery. They fear a lot of other things, real and imagined.

However, the fear of the person who has been told he is dying is a cold, clutching fear, a universally overwhelming feeling, and it strikes to the very core of his being. The fear of immediate death — through accident or assault — is physiological in nature, then it becomes emotional. However, when the threat of death is not immediate — as in a terminal diagnosis — the fear is more cerebral, more psychological, more emotional.

The fear of a "sentence of death" is universal, however much people may say they do not fear death. It is possible, however, to see the fear of one who denies his fear. It can be seen in his visual presentation, in his body language, and in reading between the lines of his conversation.

The patient had come into the hospital with cancer of the colon. When told he was terminally ill, he accepted the information calmly, saying he had no fear of dying. In fact, he made what he considered proof statements to confirm his lack of fear.

During a visit by the hospital chaplain, the patient called his visitor's attention to a book on the bedside table and asked the chaplain if he had read it. When the chaplain said he hadn't, the patient began to tell him about it. He told him that the book, which had been written by a physician, was based on the theory of treating cancer patients with a wholistic medical approach. One important aspect of this approach was the emotional support that comes with positive thinking and positive suggestion.

While the man was talking about the book and, at the same time, reaffirming his lack of fear, he was implicitly asking the chaplain if he believed what was written in the book. He wanted the chaplain to say that, yes, there was something positive about the theory. The patient's whole being was directed toward the hope in that book. The man was frightened. There was no question about it. But he would not allow himself to admit that he was frightened because it isn't macho to be afraid of things — even things that one has a right to be afraid of.

Once the fear caused by threat to the very core of the person's being has subsided, his fears become more specific. He fears the unknown related to the certainty of the prognosis. He is fearful of the changes that will take place in his body. He is fearful of the death experience itself. He also has other fears.

Often persons who are ill experience feelings of separation and isolation, even when they are being cared for at home. It is separation and isolation caused by the fact of illness — a change in routine, a change in relationships, and perhaps, a change in the person himself. Although the separation and isolation may be emotional rather than physical, these feelings come at a time when the patient is so much in need of closeness, companionship, support, and understanding from family members as well as caregivers.

A terminal diagnosis often widens the gap, temporarily or permanently, between the patient and his friends and loved ones. The enormity and depth of feelings that no one else can really understand and share isolate the dying person even more. In some ways, he is in a world of his own.

Among the feelings shared by persons who are seriously ill are feelings of helplessness and dependence. Whether the person is in the hospital or whether the person is at home, the degree of his dependence may range from minimal to total, from minimum supervision of regimen to complete and total dependence. With dependence come feelings of helplessness and powerlessness, and with these feelings often come feelings of resentment and fear of the institution or the caregiver.

For the terminally ill patient, particularly the cancer patient, the dependence finally becomes complete — as can the feelings of helplessness and powerlessness and resentment and fear. It is very important for those who care for terminally ill persons to help that person keep as much control over his life as is physically and emotionally possible. Persons who are ill have numerous concerns related to, or caused by, their illness. In general, they are concerned about their condition, about the prognosis related to their condition, about any changes in their life-style that might be required as the result of the illness. Hospital patients are usually concerned about their health, about their safety, and about the quality of services they need and receive.

One of the basic concerns of the dying patient centers on family relationships. If the family's breadwinner, he is concerned about the family's material needs and how well they will be met after his death. He is concerned about the cost of his illness and about how it will be covered. He is concerned about whether his financial affairs are in order. If the terminally ill patient is the wife and/or mother, she will be concerned about how the children will be cared for, how her husband will manage, what she can do to help prepare them to live without her.

The dying person is also usually concerned about unresolved conflicts in family relationships and about the physical and emotional toll being taken on family members and friends as a result of the illness.

John's death came after a long illness. He had been chronically ill for many, many years, and over these years, he and his wife had been at odds from time to time.

Before he died, John (with the help of his family and a counselor) was able to come to terms with the feelings they had had about him and about his chronic illness. He encouraged his wife and children to talk out some of their feelings, and he began to open up and talk about his own feelings. All of them were able, finally, to talk about and come to grips with their negative feelings about each other. When John's death came, it was very peaceful, and his family was reconciled. This brought a beautiful conclusion to what had, actually, been a beautiful and productive life.

Reconciliation is important for family members, too. Unless they have the opportunity to reconcile their differences, their ambivalence, and their conflicts with the dying person, they will have ongoing feelings of unfinished business, and feelings of unfinished business can cause long-term and unnatural grief. Patient and family members need to share and examine their feelings, do some soul searching, begin to pick up and put together the pieces of family relationships, and start the process of letting go.

Many of the needs of the dying person are very similar to those of other persons who are ill. Sometimes they vary in focus or degree. Among the dying person's most basic needs is the need to talk about his illness and death and to feel that someone understands, at least a little bit.

Because many physicians will not acknowledge that a patient is terminally ill, that patient is often denied the opportunity to talk about his illness and about what being terminally ill means to him. Too often, willingly or unwillingly, the family becomes part of this "conspiracy of silence," which hurts the family as much as the patient.

As do other patients, the dying person needs acceptance of himself as he is. This person may be, in his own eyes, less than a complete person because of loss of control over his body or because of bodily mutilation resulting from surgery or simply because he is dying.

The young woman had undergone surgery several times. Now it had become clear that she was terminally ill. Over the last few months of her life, she became reconciled with, and developed a closeness to, her philandering ex-husband. They began to be able to talk out things they had never been able to talk about before. Through this talking and sharing, the patient discovered that she could be herself, experience herself without being judged. She had achieved something she had needed so desperately — acceptance.

Not only did this young woman need acceptance — by her husband and by members of the hospital staff — she also needed that acceptance affirmed, in both words and actions. She needed to have confirmed that she was a total person, a total, feminine woman even though she was dying, and she had that confirmation.

The dying person, perhaps, needs even more acceptance and affirmation than other persons who are ill. He needs to know that he is a valuable person, no matter what his appearance, no matter what his condition, no matter how long he has to live. He needs to know that that acceptance will be confirmed for the rest of his life.

The dying person also needs empathy — not cold objectivity or unconditioned sympathy. Empathy is the midpoint between these extremes. The empathic relationship is the kind of critical (intensely self-conscious) involvement in which the person giving the care does not submerge himself into the patient's life. Instead, the caregiver maintains and protects his own identity. The empathic relationship helps fill the patient's need for understanding.

Her name was Mary, and she had come to the hospital for a neurosurgical procedure. After surgery, she had become a voiceless quadraplegic. She could see and she could hear, but she could not move and she could not talk, and she was terminally ill.

A minister who had formed an empathic relationship with Mary suggested that she use fantasy to experience things in a new way — a way that she had never experienced before. He suggested that she take fantasy trips to all of the far-off places in the world, to all of the places that she had ever wanted to visit. He reminded her that she could take these trips anytime she wanted to. That minister had given her something that no one else had been able to give her — understanding and a way out of the prison of her condition. She enjoyed those fantasy trips, and she could acknowledge them through the movement of her eyebrows and her eyelids. Every time the minister came into her room, Mary's eyes lit up like a Christmas tree. He had made waiting to die not quite so painful because he had empathy and understanding.

Another of the most basic needs of the seriously ill person, particularly the dying person, is the need for preservation of dignity and for humane and caring treatment. Hospice is the single element in the health care system in which the patient's need for dignity and caring treatment is understood, respected, and acted upon.

To die with dignity is a nearly universal wish of terminally ill patients. Making that wish come true is an important goal of hospice workers. At the end of a person's life, when a cure is not possible, he needs humane and caring treatment more than he needs the technical and practical skills of the health care practitioner.

The Right to Die

As a person's life is coming to a close, the question often arises about the person's right to die. Most often, it arises when the person's life is being sustained through professional heroics and through the miracles and marvels of medical technology.

The patient, who had a chronic illness — a type of blood cancer — entered the hospital during the last stages of his illness. After he had been there a few days, the man's physician asked his wife how long she wanted her husband to live. The physician went on to explain that with continued chemotherapy and blood transfusions her husband might live another six months. Without them, he told her gently, her husband would live only a week or two. The physician cautioned the woman, however, that if her husband's life were prolonged, he would be in and out of consciousness. He would have discomfort and he would exhibit little rational thinking or behaving. It was, he said, a matter of quality of life versus quantity of life.

The woman talked a long time with the hospital's pastoral counselor. They discussed, at great length, the decision she would have to make. Then the woman went home to think about and pray over her decision. The next morning, she called her husband's physician and told him she did not want to prolong his life with chemotherapy and blood transfusions. She opted for quality of life and for his right to die — a request he had made some time earlier.

The patient's right to die involves his right also to die with dignity — one of the most basic of all human needs — his right to let go when he is ready, and his right, if at all possible, to choose the place of his death. Too often, the "right to die" is contingent on the "permission" of the health care establishment — on the physician's willingness to recognize and accept the fact that patients do die and to accept that death is not a personal or professional affront or failure, or the failure of medicine itself.

The teacher, a brittle diabetic, had been brought to the hospital after a fall that had produced multiple fractures. The healing was painfully slow and soon her physician realized that the patient would not live very much longer.

A friend and counselor spent her last night with her. That night she talked about her feelings and about what she would have done had she had more time and more strength. She wasn't sure she was going to die that night, but she was a little depressed and she suggested that it might be her last night. The woman showed no rancor, bitterness, or fear. She was just a little bit depressed because there were so many things she would have liked to have done.

Sometime during the evening, the woman's physician stopped in to see her. She had become one of his favorites. He sat down and he talked with her and he listened to her. During their talk, the physician experienced something he had never experienced before. He found that he could talk with a dying patient without feeling that something tragic was happening. Afterwards, the physician was able to acknowledge and accept the fact that it's all right for his patients to die, that it does not represent failure.

It is in the hospice movement that a person's right to die and die with dignity are completely understood and respected.

Chapter 4

THE HOSPICE CAREGIVER

"If any lift of mine may lose
The burden of another
God give me love and care and strength
To help my ailing brother"
Anon.

BECAUSE of our original belief that hospice workers are a very special kind of people needing a special kind of training, we corresponded with five first-generation, pioneering hospice nurses across the continent. We had been given their names and told that they were sensitive, insightful, and very good at what they do. We wanted to know who they were and what made them special, and we found out.

At the time of this correspondence, there were no hospice nurse programs and no carefully drawn list of characteristics and qualifications for hospice workers, so we queried our correspondents about these things. What was your motivation for becoming a hospice nurse? What kind of experience did you have? Was it hard to go from acute-care training to hospice nursing? What are

Our correspondents were Cynthia Ishler, R.N., currently a member of the Board of Trustees of Northwest Ohio Hospice Association, Toledo, Ohio and formerly a community health nurse working in a pilot hospice home care program in Toledo, Ohio; Carolyn Jaffe, R.N., Hospice of Metro-Denver, Inc., Denver, Colorado; Noreen McNairn, R.N., B. SCN. assistant director, Hamilton-Wentworth Home Care Program, Hamilton, Ontario, Canada; Phyllis Taylor, R.N., currently with the Osteopathic Medical Center of Philadelphia, formerly Hospice Services, Death and Dying Program, Albert Einstein Medical Center, Philadelphia, Pennsylvania; and Joy Ufema, R.N., death and dying nurse, Hospice of Lancaster County, Pennsylvania.

the characteristics of a good hospice nurse? What kind of education and training is needed?

These remarkable women wrote back at length and with passion
about their motivation, about their commitment, about their
backgrounds, about their joys, frustrations, and anxieties, and
about their own needs for emotional support and renewal. The
response was overwhelming.

With grateful appreciation, we offer these insights from our
caring correspondents.

Motivation and Preparation

As early as 1973, Joy Ufema was working with terminally ill
patients in a position that she, herself, had created — death and
dying nurse. She began her work, she wrote, simply by feeling in
her heart that she had an affinity with the dying patient.

"I suppose at that time the work I was doing could have been
labeled hospice," she said. "My goal was to get the patient home
to die in his own bed, with family and community support." But
Joy conceded that she wasn't very experienced in working with
community services, so she often relied simply on the patient's
family. After an early trial-and-error start, Joy began the serious
study of the whole area of thanatology. As with most early hospice nurses, Joy was self-taught. As she wrote, "There was no mas-
ter's degree program in death and dying."

"Throughout my nursing education," wrote Cynthia Ishler, "I
was aware that people who were dying somehow didn't fit into
the activity of the hospital." Because her mother had died when
Cynthia was young, she started early in life thinking about how
death affects people. Her sensitivity to the needs of persons who
were dying led Cynthia to attend conferences on terminal care,
read extensively in the areas of terminal care and the psychological
impact of death, and to lead adult discussions on dying and its
meaning to life.

It was through her program of self-education that Cynthia
learned about the hospice concept — a concept that she understood intuitively and accepted immediately.

When Phyllis Taylor looked around after finishing nursing
school, she asked herself which categories of patients were least

wanted by society. She saw that it was "clearly those who were elderly, clearly those who were poor economically, clearly those who were dying."

"For me," she said, "the enemy is not death. The enemy is very clearly suffering. Because the enemy is not death, going into hospice work was not difficult. I was never interested in acute-care medicine per se. I worked only seven months as a staff nurse." During that time, Phyllis said, "I was so appalled by the insensitivity I saw toward patients and the judgmental care they were being given, I decided I would try teaching nursing students — particularly freshmen — so that I could work with them as their attitudes were forming.

"I was not prepared, specifically, for this type of work," Phyllis said. "I had some consulting background, some exposure to theology, and I had nurses training as well as a degree in sociology. The nursing training was helpful in terms of understanding what's going on in the body and what options people have in terms of cure, of prolonging life significantly, and of palliation. My socio-logical background and my psychological background also helped me because I had been exposed to many different kinds of people with life patterns and systems unique to their own cultures, to their own religions, and to their own ages."

"My preparation for hospice work came almost exclusively from experience," Noreen McNairn told us, "my own and those of my peers. In nursing school we learned almost nothing about the care of the dying patient, although the textbooks clearly described the process involved in tissue death. It was on the wards and in community health that my training in this field was carried out, and my best teachers were the patients and their families."

Transition and Adaptation

All of our correspondents were trained in acute-care medicine, but adapting to the new concept did not seem to present a real problem for any of them.

"My personality was not that of an acute-care nurse," wrote Joy Ufema. "I did not prefer emergency room nursing and card-ioverting and that stressful, quick-thinking-on-your-feet type of nursing. That is not my style. And I think it's imperative for all of us, whatever work we do, to feel in our hearts that we're good at something and that we do a good job at that task."

"Having been an intensive care nurse," wrote Carolyn Jaffe, "I found the transition easy." Carolyn referred to the evolution of her own philosophy regarding care of the terminal patient, as it came to fit the hospice model.

Making the transition from acute care to hospice care has a lot to do with redefining success, wrote Cynthia Ishler. "In community health, as in the hospital, the nurse's goal is to assist the client to reach a level of wellness so that he or she no longer needs nursing assistance. When the person is discharged from the hospital, or the record is closed, the goal has been reached and the nurse is successful. In hospice, the family needs assistance through the dying process and beyond. So, in hospice care, there must be different criteria for defining success."

Cynthia also wrote that it is necessary, although sometimes difficult, to sort out important tasks from less important ones. "An example comes to mind," she wrote. "Another nurse in our agency was caring for a man who was terminally ill, who could not eat. The nurse was frantically trying dietary supplements and having the family experiment with techniques for feeding." According to Cynthia, the client was not uncomfortable nor did he complain of hunger. Even so, the nurse did not seem to be able to accept the fact that it was not her responsibility to keep the man alive by forcing him to eat. She had "lost sight of the quality versus quantity thinking."

Although the transition from acute care to hospice care was not very difficult for her, Noreen McNairn commented thoughtfully, "Because almost all health professionals have their training geared toward goals of making people better, it is always difficult to stand by and see a patient deteriorate despite your efforts. We as caregivers still tend to fight too long to 'cure' someone. As a result, we are sometimes unable to help a patient and family to accept a terminal diagnosis because we are unable to accept this ourselves."

Emotional Support

The need for emotional support was on the minds of the nurses who wrote to us.

As Cynthia Ishler said, society, by and large, has a hard time understanding someone who cares for dying patients. Non-hospice nurses often do not understand and do not want to listen to the hospice nurse.

However, the need for sharing their feelings is great among hospice nurses. Someone with "an understanding heart" is the way Noreen McNairn described the kind of person who can provide emotional support for hospice caregivers. The person who has knowledge and experience together with the ability to listen without making judgements and to experience empathy without the obstruction of emotional involvement is needed.

"It is essential to me," said Noreen, "that I have someone with whom I can share my personal frustrations regarding palliative care. It is usually one of our social workers with whom I share my feelings." This person, Noreen said, is one who maintains an objective viewpoint and directs her thoughts toward partial and sometimes complete solutions.

"A caring life mate — one who can listen and comment maturely and objectively," is Carolyn Jaffe's source of emotional support.

"I think we get into trouble," wrote Joy Ufema, "trying to be stoic super-nurses. I feel the secret to being able to stay in this work and not burn out is to be real at all times. When I am feeling sad and overwrought with work or death, I express those feelings. I grieve a great deal and express that grief through crying. I express it through going to funerals, which I think is imperative so that I have a sense of closure about the relationship. Personally, I have one or two friends with whom I can be real and with whom I am very safe to say, 'I'm tired and I need help for a while.' "

"My need," wrote Cynthia Ishler, "is to talk about what is happening to the families and what that's doing to me. Talking helps get everything into perspective. I had several close friends who accepted, if not truly understood, how I was feeling. These people would let me talk about dying as much as I needed to. They understood why I enjoyed my work." (One of the hardest things for a person to understand is how anyone can enjoy hospice work.)

"Emotional support comes from a variety of people," Phyllis Taylor told us. "There have been some lovely people I have worked with who have been very supportive. My husband and my children have been supportive also. But I must say, it takes a tremendous toll on people who do this work and on their families. I found that I *could not and should not* rely on my family as my main base of emotional support."

Most of these nurses told us that other members of the hospice team provide most of their emotional support. Said Carolyn Jaffe, "those who do this work understand and are able to listen and hear at the time you need support."

But it's not enough, they said, to share feelings and cares and frustrations. It is important, they wrote, to have adequate time away from work and to have activities that help them relax and have fun — to experience personal renewal.

Personal Characteristics

Our correspondents wrote about the personal characteristics needed in being an effective and fulfilled hospice worker. They ranged from flexibility to a sense of humor. They included respect, patience, maturity, commitment, confidence, and love. They also included having the ability to share openly, knowing one's own strengths and weaknesses, and having come to terms with death — being comfortable with dying.

Most of the nurses talked in terms of having some conviction about belief in the existence of a God. "I do have a religious conviction," said Joy Ufema. "I find that almost imperative in dealing with death and dying." Even so, Joy said her hospice volunteers can be atheists. "I just want them to be very firm in their religion or in their lack of religion."

In a similar vein, Carolyn Jaffe had this to say, "I think it's most important to have some feeling of believing in God — independent of religion. One must be able to go into a person's home, as a guest, and relate to their religious beliefs, to be understanding and worldy, to pray with them if they ask, but at no time to infringe on their privacy."

"I'm Jewish," said Phyllis Taylor, "but I'm a Quaker theologically. Because of the Jewish background I have a focus on family unit, on the need for that, and an acute awareness of how life is made up not only of joy but also of suffering. The Quaker part of me is the part that enables me to see all people as completely equal, no matter what their economic status, racial status, or nationality status. I go to Meeting for Worship and I've found that the times sitting quietly in Meeting for Worship have been very helpful to me in terms of renewal. There is an absolute passion that sustains me. I think that passion comes from God."

According to Phyllis, personal qualities needed by hospice workers include compassion, a sense of justice, steadfastness, patience. It also takes a sense of advocacy, she said, a willingness to really listen, the ability to suspend your own judgments, and the ability to see who the enemy is — to decide that the enemy isn't death but suffering and then to go after that suffering.

Finally, Noreen McNairn wrote that the hospice worker needs to "be able to listen without judgment, able to weep without guilt, able to guide without pressure, and able to share feelings without shame."

Satisfactions

In openly sharing their satisfactions and frustrations, these hospice nurses wrote both about the rewards of relationships and the frustration of the existing system.

"I'm always satisfied," said Noreen McNairn, "when I have helped a patient and family to adjust to an altered mode of living and I feel the same way when I am able to be a part of the support for a patient and family prior to and after death. I suppose that the satisfaction comes when you have heard a patient say that he is grateful for having been allowed to share those very important final months or days together at home. Maybe," she continued, "we should express our thanks to these families for allowing us to share with them these very special times."

"I guess I've always been a scrapper," Joy Ufema wrote. "I enjoy fighting for the underdog and, certainly, I feel that the dying patient is that. I guess it's also because I have a vested interest. I, too, must die and it matters to me how I die. I want to have a good death that takes place in my own bed with my cats and dogs and horses surrounding me."

"The fulfillment," said Phyllis Taylor, "is seeing someone who is physically pain free, who is able to communicate with his family, and who's been able to make decisions about where he or she wants to be and how he or she wants to live his life — whether that's for a day or a week or a month. I have found that each person is so totally individualized that you cannot impose your preconceptions on them. It took me a while to realize that each person is going through dying in his own way — not Elisabeth Kubler-Ross' way or in my way or in anybody else's way, but uniquely in his own way.

Satisfaction is in knowing that when he dies he did it in his own way and in knowing that, as family members rebuild their own emotions and their own lives without the person who has just died, they won't have so many 'if onlys' that I hear so often from people who have not had hospice support. People are haunted by 'if onlys.' "

"There were lots of things that made me enjoy hospice care," said Cynthia Ishler. "I feel that dealing with dying is never easy, but I think hospice makes it less difficult. Being able to enter a home and help readjust schedules and medications, so that the family was less chaotic and the client more comfortable, was very satisfying. Helping people deal with a situation that seemed impossible and seeing them be successful made the effort worthwhile."

"Hospice," said Carolyn Jaffe, "fulfills an insatiable need of mine to help, to be needed, and to please."

"Job satisfaction is wonderful when I can do my job well," Phyllis Taylor told us. "The medical system is so much a disease-oriented system and hospice care, in so many ways, is such a life-oriented system that they often clash. I see this in the acute-care setting where you work and work and work to get someone pain-controlled and then have it all fall to pieces because a post-operative patient comes up at ten to twelve. The hospice patient should have had medication at twelve, but doesn't get the medication until quarter of one. The patient is back in pain and back in the pain cycle."

"My own frustrations," wrote Noreen McNairn," are created by the red tape — the incredible web woven by our progressive society in which we all become entangled. There are the hospitals who have the right to refuse the admission of a patient if there is no treatment goal. There are rules about the needless intervention of a coroner in some instances. There are physicians who do not feel they can cope with the responsibility of caring for a patient and family once all hope for recovery is gone. There are, most of all, the attitudes of health professionals who refuse to recognize the right of a patient to refuse treatment and to die without further medical intervention."

Cynthia Ishler, having been away from hospice work for almost a year, considered the question of concerns and frustrations. "I remember most of the positive and very little of the negative feelings I had. Near the end of my time with hospice, however, I was a classic case of burnout. A lot of it was a feeling of lack of support administratively.

"A major concern was always acceptance by the medical community, primarily physicians. They were always very much in agreement with the concept, but they were either unwilling to give the dying patient the time he required or none of *their* patients were terminal. (But hospice was a good idea for those who *were* terminal.)"

For Phyllis Taylor, the biggest frustration is seeing people suffer unnecessarily and not having the credentials to prescribe adequate medication — even though she has a better sense than many physicians of the hospice philosophy concerning pharmacological pain management. "I could make recommendations, but I could not write orders. That was the kind of frustration I had. It was not the orientation of 'save life at any cost,' which is what you are trained to do in the acute-care setting.

"Frustration is seeing needs and not being able to meet them because I don't have the power to meet them, and it's very much a question of power. Another frustration is that in nursing schools and medical schools, there still are not enough programs that deal with the terminally ill person through a life-oriented focus. There are very few programs that deal with good pain management.

"Yet another frustration is seeing physicians unable to let go enough to say, 'My goal is no longer to cure the person, no longer to prolong the person's life significantly. My goal is good palliation.' Most physicians still can't understand that concept, I find, and many nurses can't either — although nurses are way ahead of physicians."

Education and Training

More than highly specialized and procedural formal education programs, the consensus is that hospice students need a program in which they can learn about death and dying and about the very special needs — emotional, spiritual, and psychosocial — of the terminally ill patient and his family. They need a program in which they learn about pain control and symptom control in an environment in which drug addiction is not a major concern.

But, as importantly, according to the nurses who wrote to us, they need a program in which they can explore and come to grips with their own attitudes toward dying and a program through which they can develop communications, counseling, and interpersonal skills to prepare them for the very human, personal, and intense relationships they will be involved in. They also need hands-on experience with a hospice program.

Training for hospice work should be a "very wholistic kind of training," said Phyllis Taylor, "training that would include theology, that would include pharmacology, that would include knowledge of disease systems, that would include cultural analysis, and that would include training for really good listening skills." Incorporating life experience is also important, Phyllis said, as is a passionate sense of justice.

Rehabilitation training would also be helpful, Phyllis told us, "I really view hospice work as a kind of rehabilitation medicine. In rehab, you're maximizing whatever potential the patient still has. In good hospice care, you're maximizing each day the potential the person has left, so that people can be maximally living while their bodies are dying."

"The training needed is not one that dwells on procedures and policies," said Noreen McNairn, "but rather one that helps us gain personal insight into our own attitudes about dying. I find it difficult to see a specific curriculum in this regard, but would anticipate benefits from having skilled counselors available, on a one-to-one basis, to discuss reactions, interactions, and plans with the student who is dealing with a dying patient. After all, the basic concept is not just to acquire knowledge, but also to make effective use of such knowledge."

According to Carolyn Jaffe, "Technical nursing experience is useful, but because the hospice nurse must most often function independently in the patient's home, the security to make good decisions and to act upon them often needs to take precedence over nursing skills."

Cynthia Ishler had a similar view. "The condition of the hospice patient can change rapidly and the nurse must have enough skill and confidence to deal almost automatically with these changes. But first of all, the nurse must be comfortable with the tasks needed to provide patient care — carrying out treatment plans, regulation of medications, and making physical assessments."

Aside from these skills, Cynthia said, "The hospice student needs training in communication and interpersonal skills." The last area, Cynthia wrote, is the area of pain control and symptom control. She put this area last, she said, not because it was the least important, but because these techniques are easy to learn. "However long it takes," Cynthia wrote, "the hospice nurse needs a solid foundation of fundamental skills."

All of our correspondents agreed that many of the skills and attitudes needed are not acquired through formal education programs but have been and can be acquired through personal education.

Despite our original premise that the type of person and the type of preparation for hospice work were of equal importance, we have learned that personal qualities and individual commitments, at this point, have a greater effect than the carefully developed and highly specialized curriculums. The modern nursing curriculum can easily — if it does not already do so — incorporate courses in palliative care, psychology, and human relations. It cannot, however, turn every young woman or young man into a caring and coping hospice nurse.

Hospice work is bittersweet, Phyllis Taylor told us. "Clearly there's tremendous bitterness in the rages of the illness — physically, financially, and psychically — but I know that there can be a lot of sweetness in terms of tremendous amounts of love and honesty and in terms of the ability to cry together as well as to laugh together."

Then Phyllis reminded us of Ecclesiastes 3:

> For everything there is a season,
>   And a time for every purpose under heaven;
> A time to be born, and a time to die;
>   A time to weep, and a time to laugh;
> A time to rend, and a time to sew;
>   A time to keep silence, and a time to speak.

Part II
HOSPICE: Some Perspectives

SEEING hospice through the eyes of those most intimately involved took us into homes, hospitals, and offices for interview after interview.

We talked for hours with individuals who were hospice founders, coordinators, program directors, physicians, nurses, social workers, and volunteers. They told us what draws them to hospice work and what that work means to them. We talked to hospice teams and learned how they work together and how they support each other.

We also talked with a young woman whose mother had received hospice care, with a man whose sister was cared for by a hospice, and with a woman who became a hospice volunteer after a serious illness that she thought was terminal. Through them, we saw hospice from yet another perspective.

All of these people talked to us with candor, with commitment, and with caring sensitivity. Here are their stories told in their own words.

Chapter 5

"THEY GOT US THROUGH IT"

DIALOGUE WITH A DAUGHTER

Cindy Mitchell is a young Chicago wife and mother who commuted to Albuquerque, N.M. for the last year of her mother's life. For six months of the last year, Cindy Mitchell's mother received home hospice care. It was provided by Hospital Home Health Care/Hospice of St. Joseph's and Presbyterian Hospitals, a program that was founded in December 1977. Cindy Mitchell recounts here the experience that her family had with hospice care.

C M   My mother had cancer. And she was in a wheelchair. She had had it, I would say, for about two or three years, and she was getting progressively worse.

       When she was young, 28 or 30, she had had a mastectomy. So she knew that she had cancer when her leg problem started. But the doctors told her that she was a hypochondriac, that she had arthritis. Then they told her she had a slipped disc, or something, and they put her in the hospital for a . . . what is that test they do on the back? . . . a myelogram.

       And she said, "Alright, you can give me the myelogram, but I won't sign any form until you promise to give me a bone scan." So the doctor, to humor her, gave her the bone scan. By that time, the cancer was in five places.. It was in the early part of 1975 that she had the myelogram and the bone scan.

R H   Then she knew that she had cancer for about five years before she died. Was she in pain a good deal of that time?

53

C M She always said she didn't have pain. And she absolutely refused to take any painkillers at all. I think that may have been, first of all, because physically she had never reacted well to any kind of strong drug. I think she took a tranquilizer once and became violently ill.

I know that she must have been in pain sometimes, but I don't think she was in terrible pain. There must be something in certain people what causes them not to have as much pain. But she never complained of pain.

R H So she really didn't suffer?

C M No . . . I don't know whether it was mind control or what. The cancer was in her hips, her legs, everywhere . . . just everywhere. There was probably a malignancy in the brain, although it never showed up in the scan. But they did find two tumors back in the . . . ah lumbar region . . . somewhere back there. They diagnosed her condition as Bell's Palsy, which it sure wasn't. It turned out to be a complete loss of muscle control on one side of her face.

She had probably had cancer for five years before it was correctly diagnosed.

R H How did you happen to become involved with a hospice program?

C M My mother very much wanted to stay at home. (Other than one short hospital stay, she was at home the whole time.) We very much appreciated her wish to stay home and we understood it. Hospitals are very cold, sterile, frightening places.

My mother loved her home and it was a beautiful home. She had a lot of beautiful things. It was her home and she wanted to keep taking care of it. She had a responsibility.

And so we decided to care for mother at home.

R H How did her doctor feel about that?

C M Oh, he supported us keeping her at home. He said, "It's your decision. If you feel that you can deal with it, I think it's a good idea." Towards the end, though, he wasn't around to hold our hands, or anything like that.

About six months prior to her death, our doctor suggested the hospice program. By this time, Mother was almost bedridden, not totally, but almost. And we were beginning to have problems in terms of things like helping her to go to the bathroom. She was also on oxygen. For some very practical reasons, and because the doctor felt that emotional support would be beneficial, he suggested the hospice.

R H   Were you and your family receptive to the idea?

C M   Oh yes, we very happily agreed to do this. We were thrilled. I may be wrong, but I think my sister Jennifer had actually looked into hospices sometime earlier. And she had talked about having some sort of support system even before that.

R H   Was your mother cared for by a hospice team?

C M   Yes. The team was divided up according to functions, so to speak. There were Nancy and Susan, who were registered nurses. At first they came every other day; later they came more often. Susan and Nancy brought a lot of fun into our house. Then there was a woman who came in every day. I believe she was an LPN or something. She provided the physical care for my mother. And, up until the last two or three months, a therapist would come in to help mother with muscle movement and things like that. So, basically, the team included the physician, who was more or less a part of it, the two nurses, the physical therapist, and the LPN.

We fired the LPN. She just did not fit into our household. She was too rigid. She didn't do well at all. The final blow-up came when she told my youngest sister that she and her friends were making too much noise in the house. That did it. My father told her to leave.

Although Mother had total care from the hospice team, we very much wanted to be part of that care. For some reason, doing things like working with the oxygen tanks made us feel very helpful. So we helped with the physical care all we could.

R H   Were Susan and Nancy available 24 hours a day?

C M   Yes, though they were each on a set schedule, we could call them any time. I'm sure there were some instances toward the end that they both came on days other than their appointed days. It seemed like they were always there. They were our strength.

R H   How long did your mother receive hospice care?

C M   About six months.

R H   How much of that time was the family able to be together?

C M   Well, during those last six months, either my sister would be there or I would be there. Then, at the end, our husbands were there too.

Earlier on, as my mother got progressively worse, my sister and I would try to go back to Albuquerque for three weeks, four times a year. Jennifer would come in from South America or Europe, wherever she was living at the time. And I would go to Albuquerque from Chicago. We tried never to have a period of more than a month when one of us wasn't there.

It was tiring and very expensive, but it was something we both wanted to do. And our husbands were very supportive.

R H   What kind of a relationship did your mother have with members of the hospice team?

C M   Mother and Susan and Nancy, especially, became very close. They had a lot of fun together and they talked about a lot of things. My mother was the kind that had just tons of friends. She drew people around her all the time. She was a very neat lady.

Susan and Nancy ended up telling my mom about their problems, which my mother loved, because she was reciprocating. She was needed. Susan would sit on the bed and talk to Mom. I guess that she came from a kind of strange situation, a strange family life in London. She used to tell my mom about these things and about her husband and she would ask Mom's advice on things. And that was wonderful. My mother always loved to be needed and to be involved in other people's lives. She'd worry about Nancy and Susan and ask them how things were going.

My mother had a terrific sense of humor. And so did Susan and Nancy. This resulted in a lot of laughter, a lot of fun, and a lot of closeness. Susan and Nancy encouraged us all to congregate in my mother's bedroom. And we'd talk and we'd laugh, and we'd do very normal, natural, fun kinds of things. Things that you wouldn't expect to do in this kind of situation. None of us had been through an experience like this. We were a very, very close family and we'd never experienced someone's death before.

Nancy and Susan got us through it. They did it in little ways. For example, Nancy would take us to lunch, if we'd had a hard morning. The three of us — Dad and Nancy and I — would go out and have a nice lunch. We'd talk about anything and everything and we'd have a good time. Sometimes we'd go over to Nancy's house and visit.

We became involved in their lives, too. We knew all about Nancy's new house, about problems with her husband's job, and about conflicts in her family. And we knew the same things about Susan. We got to know their husbands. We still see them. In fact, at Christmastime, we had Susan and her husband over for a party. And my dad still sees Nancy. We became very close to these people. Very much so.

R H Would you say that it was to your advantage that you became this close?

C M To our advantage? Yes. To their advantage? Probably not. But very much to our advantage.

I don't think that you would be effective if you didn't have that involvement. I know that we, personally, were looking for that kind of emotional support. We needed to have someone to talk to that was understanding and compassionate. And I don't think you can have those qualities without involvement.

But the involvement was hard on Nancy. I know that the day after my mother died, and for a few days afterward, she took off work. She had trouble dealing with it. It hurt her a lot. They became very close.

R H You said earlier that you were involved in your mother's physical care. Why was that important to you?

C M Why was it important? We felt very proud. I was extremely proud that I had learned how to handle the big oxygen tanks we had in the closet. I had learned how to turn off one tank, disconnect it, and connect the other one. I also learned how to keep the oxygen tank at the right level.

Nancy also showed us how to put a . . . some kind of thing for the bladder . . . a balloon-like thing . . .

R H   A catheter.

C M   Right, it was a catheter. If something had happened that made her unable to urinate, we had been instructed on how to put a catheter in her. Fortunately, we didn't have to do this. But we knew how. We also administered Librium® and some kind of pill she was on up until very close to the end. It was a pill given in the chemotherapy that she had — not a painkiller by any means. We kept charts of her medicine, too.

During the evening, we did all of the bathroom stuff. And we alternated so that my dad could get a rest. Jennifer would take one time and I would take another. We would lift her onto the toilet and we took care of all of her physical needs. And there were times when it was hard. But we wanted to do it.

I think Mom's death would have been a thousand times worse if we hadn't had been involved in that way. It must be a very frightening thing to have somebody die in a hospital where you have no contact with them and no physical involvement. I think that would be very, very hard.

R H   Was part of your reason for wanting to be involved in your mother's physical care the need to keep busy?

C M   Oh, no! We kept ourselves busy. That wasn't it. It was absolutely an emotional involvement.

R H   You've talked about the involvement of Nancy and Susan in your mother's care. What about the physician's involvement?

C M   We didn't see much of him towards the end. He would bop in for two minutes and that was it. He was an excellent doctor, but he had a tendency not to tell us what was happening. It was Susan and Nancy who would talk to us if we were having problems. They'd make us feel better. And they would also honestly explain to us everything that was happening, which the doctor didn't do.

I remember one thing the doctor did that really irritated us. Mom had gone into a coma (two or three days before she died) and standing in her room, the doctor said, "She's dying." Well we knew she was dying, but he said it in a rather cruel way. Then he said, "She's in a coma and she can't hear anything you say." My dad was standing by Mom's bed and he saw tears coming down her face. We thought that was an incredible thing to say. She really liked this doctor.

Maybe this was an example of someone who didn't want to get involved. I mean, it must be terrible to be a cancer specialist, which he was. I guess you lose a lot of patients. After a certain point, he had showed no emotion. He bopped in and he bopped out. He made that little comment. And we never saw him again.

When he made that comment about not hearing what we said, we thought, "baloney!" We spent a lot of time talking with her and she heard us. My mother always talked with her eyebrows. It was very expressive the way her eyebrows went up and down. One time when we were in her room talking about something and laughing, we noticed her eyebrows going up and down. And just four hours before she died, she squeezed my hand very tightly.

R H What would you have hoped the doctor would have done during that last visit?

C M I think if he had said just one little thing. If he had said, "Well, we tried. I enjoyed knowing her." If he had just showed . . . you know . . . some feeling. But it was like Mom had become a nonentity. And I think we all resented that. I don't think it's right for the family or the patient.

R H Do you think maybe he felt a sense of failure?

C M We all thought that. It's definitely one possibility . . . that he couldn't deal with failure or that he has, in fact, built up some sort of facade, which may very well be necessary. I don't think I could do it. I don't know.

R H How much before your Mother's death did you accept the fact that she was dying?

C M   I think that we knew from day one. Jennifer and I did at least.

R H   Day one, meaning the six months of hospice care?

C M   No. I mean the day that we found out she had cancer.

R H   Five years before?

C M   Yes, because the cancer was just everywhere. In fact, the doctor told us, at some point toward the end, that he hadn't expected her to live for six months. She had holes in the bones of both hips. And she had cancer in her lungs.

I think Jennifer and I accepted it from the beginning, but hoped and prayed that she would live a long time. Of course we would grasp at any little positive kind of thing, but I don't think either of us thought she would recover. Jen and I talked between ourselves constantly about it and we, in turn, acted as support for our younger sister.

I don't think my mother accepted it and I think it was positive that she didn't. She fought to the very end.

Dad was the slowest to accept it. He is a very religious person and I think he really believed for a long time that by some kind of miracle, or whatever, my mother wouldn't die. We didn't realize that for a long time. He was always optimistic with us. We always thought he was doing it for Mother's benefit and for our benefit. Towards the end, however, we realized that he was saying what he really believed.

It was Nancy who sat down in the living room with him one day and said, "Matt, she's going to die." She helped him become aware of the reality. I think the finality of the whole thing stunned him.

R H   How long before your mother died did Nancy talk with him?

C M   Maybe two, maybe three weeks before. None of us realized until that point what he had been doing. We thought he was just being the very strong, optimistic person that was going to carry us all the way through this. Then we realized that he was just denying what we had accepted months ago.

R H   You said Susan and Nancy were your strength and your support.

C M   In terms of emotional support, they were unbelievable. Without the support they gave us, it would have been a very frightening experience. Nancy explained each step to us.

R H   You mean each physical step?

C M   Each physical step, yes. She told us everything that was happening and why it was happening. She told us not to be afraid, that this thing was normal and that it wasn't a sign of pain. She explained to us as we progressed what to expect, so when it did happen, we weren't shocked and weren't afraid.

R H   She was preparing you.

C M   Oh, absolutely. I think she started four or five days before, telling us little bits . . . you know . . . there would be labored breathing. And when that started, we should call her right away, which we did. She came instantly. And she told us other things to expect — but in a very unfrightening way. Then once we were actually involved in my mother's dying — we were all there — she told us the next thing that might happen. "If such and such happens," she said, "don't be afraid. It's normal. She's not in pain." We'd ask a question and we'd get a very honest answer.

R H   Did your mother agree to hospice care because she accepted the fact that she was going to die or did she agree to it because she didn't want to go to the hospital?

C M   I think it was an acceptance of *care* as well as not wanting to go to the hospital. I guess the one thing that we were not successful in doing — if that's the way to put it — was in talking with her about her acceptance of death.

       She never really, sincerely said, "I'm going to die," until about two weeks before she died. She would say, from time to time, "I'm not going to get over this." I think, for her, we did the right thing. We'd say "yeh, yeh, you'll get over this," because she was a fighter and that's what kept her going on as long as she did. And for her it was right. She kept fighting until the very, very end.

R H   Would it have helped you or your mother if you had been able to talk about her death?

C M   Maybe at the end, but I don't think so before, because she was going to fight. At the end, I think it would have helped, but unfortunately the last five or six weeks, the so-called Bell's Palsy caused such a severe problem that she had trouble speaking. Once it started happening, her condition deteriorated rapidly to the point that it was difficult for her to make long sentences. It was hard for her to talk and she would get so mad.

Her mind was working fine, although there were times when she was hallucinating. She just couldn't get the words out. She made kind of a sputtering sound. And she couldn't get the words out. Oh, she got so furious, but in a very funny way.

R H   I'm a little bit surprised. Normally, a person like your mother would be told she was dying.

C M   For my mother, I'm not sure it would have been right.

R H   I've gone through this with families so many times. The family's afraid that knowing is going to make the dying person upset. But let me give you an example . . .

C M   You know, you've rung a bell with me. When I say my mother never admitted it . . . and I haven't talked about this in a long time . . . I'm wrong. We did talk about it in a strange kind of way, I guess.

We talked about what she wanted to wear. She told me months before what dress she wanted to wear and how she wanted to look. I can't believe that I had forgotten all of this.

Five or six months before, she had made out her will. She kept saying, "I want to write out a will." And I kept saying, "eeeehhhh," which was a mistake on my part. And than I said to myself, "That's stupid. She wants to do this."

We had a wonderful evening. She had me bring into her bedroom every single thing in the house that was special to her. And we got out all of her jewelry and looked at it and talked about it. We really had a good time. I can remember sitting up late that night. And it was . . . it was enjoyable. We remembered who gave her each piece and whether it was my grandmother's.

We wrote it all down and we talked about her dying. I sat up with her until midnight.

R H How do you think other people would have thought about your talking this way?

C M My sister, who was not there, but was coming into the country shortly, was thrilled that it had happened.

Jennifer had wanted us to have some kind of death counseling. She had been very adamant about that. But my dad — and now I realize why — didn't want to do it.

But we did talk about it, Mother and I . . . about her death. Maybe it's because we talked about it in such a pleasant way that I didn't remember it and maybe because only once did she cry and say, "I'm going to die."

R H What happened when she did die? Were you relieved that she was no longer suffering?

C M Because of the hallucinations toward the end, I don't think that I could say that we were relieved that her suffering was over. I think I can say, and I want to explain this, that we were relieved that our suffering was over. Because it was time.

R H And you were all hurting.

C M And we were all hurting. At the end, she just couldn't eat. We had been feeding her for some time, but it was all coming back up. So the doctor told us to stop feeding her because she would choke.

My dad asked if we could put her on intravenous feeding. And the four of us — my dad and Jennifer and Carrie and I — went into the living room and talked about it. Jennifer and Carrie and I said, "No, let's don't prolong this. Let's just let nature take its course." It was a conscious decision. All we could have done was to have her hooked up to a machine and we never even considered that.

R H And Susan and Nancy supported you in this decision?

C M Gosh, yes. They prepared us. And Nancy was with us through the whole thing.

Mom died on my birthday. I think we all knew that was going to be the day. But she didn't die until evening. Even though she was in a coma, I think that she wanted to make sure that she stayed alive until my birthday, so that we could all sit on her bed and open presents like we had done for 30 years.

It was a strange day. You know, no matter how well you plan for something, things go wrong? Well, my husband Stephen and I had borrowed his father's car to go out to the airport to pick up my sister's husband. We stopped by his mother and father's house and his mother said we had better get home. After we got to my parent's home, Stephen's father called and said, "I need my car." So Steve had to leave.

I needed his support. I needed him there. During the time he was gone, my mother died. And it was hard on me, harder for just a moment than I thought it would be. But a minute later, Mom started to breathe again, in a very raspy, terrifying kind of way. In about 20 minutes, Steve came back in. And Mom's whole body became very calm. And she died very quietly and very calmly.

I think — and we convinced ourselves — that she could view this whole scene and she realized that I needed additional support. Who knows.

R H   You're saying that you felt she came back.

C M   Yes. I felt that way very strongly! I think it was an incredible help. There was some other incident that day. Something very strange but I don't remember exactly what it was. There were all these little things that we felt at the time. And emotionally I think it was good for us to feel the way we did.

R H   What happened immediately after she died?

C M   Well, after it was all over and they had come for the body, we all went into the kitchen because we were all absolutely starving. Nancy walked into the kitchen and she had a birthday cake for me. And that was nice. There we were, eating and drinking coffee and having birthday cake. And we had a nice evening. That sounds sort of awful, doesn't it?

R H   Why do you think it sounds awful?

C M   Well, I think you always have this preconceived notion that death is going to be very tearful and . . .

R H And your hospice experience changed that?

C M Oh, yes! It took our fear away for one thing, particularly during the time my mother was dying. I think that for someone who had never been through the experience before to go through it at home without this kind of support would be very frightening. As Mom's condition worsened, Nancy explained everything to us.

R H How did your family respond to your mother's death?

C M I think in as healthy a way as possible. My middle sister, the one in Germany, responded in much the same way as I did. In a lot of ways, my youngest sister had the most difficulty. She was just sixteen when my mother became ill. So she took the brunt of it. We were a very, very close family and had always had a lot of fun together. And I think Carrie felt that she'd been denied the kind of family relationship that Jennifer and I had had at that age. I think she had problems with it, but with the support of the family and everyone else involved, she wound up doing fine. My dad took it very well.

R H Did Nancy and Susan attend the funeral?

C H Oh yes. My two sisters and I did the eulogy and we, basically, conducted the funeral. That was the way it should be. We did everything the way we wanted to. No matter what the funeral director said. It was a very personal and a very nice service. We felt such pride when it was all over, because we did it. We did it the way we wanted to do it and the way she wanted it done.

After the funeral, we gave a very large party and invited all of our friends. Nancy and Susan and their husbands came. And we all had a very good time.

Epilogue

R H Cindy, you cried a few minutes ago.

C M My mother was really the most incredible woman I have ever known. It's still hard for me to talk about.

R H Why is it difficult for you to talk about?

C M Because I loved her very much. Such a neat lady!

R H   What happens when you celebrate your birthday?

C M   In the beginning I worried about that. I thought, "Boy, my birthday is going to be awful for the rest of my life." And it isn't. It's just not. My mother's death passes through my mind, obviously. Sometimes I'll find that it'll pass through my mind in the first part of February and I'll come to dread my birthday. And then, sometimes, I'll honestly forget.

On my birthday, my dad and my sisters and I get on the phone and talk. We always do on our birthdays. We mention the subject, of course, but it isn't like the celebration of a tragedy or anything like that.

R H   How is your father doing now?

C M   At first he was very lonely, because my younger sister married a year after my mother died. So he sold our home and moved to an apartment. He was lonely there, too. Now, though he still has periods of loneliness, he's doing very well.

R H   He must be dating again.

C M   Yeh. And it's great with us. My dad, who is 75, is now taking a driving tour around the country with a 35-year-old woman from Thailand. And I love it that he's having a good time. I wish this would happen every day.

R H   What about Nancy and Susan?

C M   Both of them have left the program. They've left hospice work altogether. I don't remember why and I should. I just saw Susan two months ago.

Both Susan and Nancy had children. And both of them felt the strain not only of the emotional involvement, but also of the time commitment, the strange hours, and being on call, basically, 24 hours a day.

R H   How do you feel about your hospice experience three years later?

C M   It was a wonderful thing. I suppose maybe it isn't for everybody. I imagine that a lot has to do with the patient's attitude and whether that person has a strong and close family. But if the patient has the right attitude and the desire and a close family, I think it would be a very serious mistake not to have hospice care. Death is an incredibly hard and hurting kind of thing to go through, but the hospice sure made it a lot easier for us.

I came home from Albuquerque and I wanted to share with all my friends what a meaningful time it had been. And share the support we had had and the way we had done it. But I found out that a lot of them really didn't want to hear. They didn't want to listen and they didn't understand. So I didn't talk about it as much as I wanted to. That's why Jennifer wrote the article on hospice. We had to tell people that there is another way to die. But I don't think anybody really cared.

Chapter 6

"IT WAS AN INNOCENT BEGINNING"

DIALOGUE WITH A HOSPICE FOUNDER

Wife of a doctor, mother of four daughters, consummate volunteer, and founder of Horizon Hospice. That's a thumbnail sketch of Ada Addington, who is a founder of the first hospice in Chicago. In the dialogue that follows, she describes how a group of four established the program, what problems they faced, how their program works, and what their plans for the future are.

R H What made you get involved in founding a hospice?

A A I have long been interested in medical things. So I started reading some articles — five or six years ago — about the hospice movement. About the idea of the hospice, which I had never heard of before six years ago. At that time, a good friend of mine, Sharon Bunyon King, a young lawyer, was also very interested in the idea. She had a medical background, too. So one day we said, "Wouldn't it be a good idea to start something like that in Chicago?" At that point, there were no such services for the terminally ill or their families in the city of Chicago. So we decided to try to begin one. I have to say that it was a very innocent beginning.

R H How did you get it started?

A A Sharon and I were joined quickly by a young pediatrician, Frank Duda, who had dealt with terminally ill children for many years and knew Elisabeth Kubler-Ross. He had worked with her and had gone to some workshops with her. There was also an Episcopalian minister, Father Wilson Reed, who was very interested in the idea of hospice. So the four of us started to read and started to gather some more interested people around us. We made visits throughout the country to various hospices.

It was at this point that we formed the board and incorporated ourselves. We went through the beginning organizational things that one has to do, which we really didn't know much about. In fact, we knew nothing about them, because none of us had ever done anything like this before. It took us a while. I think probably one of the most difficult things we did was to write a proposal — a grant proposal — which none of us had ever done either. It forced us to clarify our thinking about what we wanted to do and what we did not want to do.

It took us a year and a half to go all through this organizational process. It was also a learning period, during which we really solidified our philosophy — although it has changed from time to time as we've progressed. I think that period was a vital one for us. We met every week in my living room for these discussions, conversations, and exchanges of ideas. This helped us enormously, because when the time came that we were ready for patients, we had an idea about what we were going to do. Quite a clear idea.

We decided to start with home care. Originally, we wanted a building right away. We wanted an inpatient unit, but little by little we discovered that that was not feasible at that time. So we switched our emphasis to home care. And you have to remember that in 1978, there was no such thing as a hospice in Chicago. However, there were a lot of people who were interested in the idea, so we quickly attracted a great many people who were very helpful to us. We formed a kind of nucleus. We had no trouble attracting volunteers or seed money in the beginning. We worked hard for it, but it was there. The interest was there.

R H   What were some of the problems you encountered?

A A   I think one of the main problems we encountered was a lack of knowledge among medical professionals about what a hospice is, about the whole idea of hospice. Most people had never heard of it. We had to spend a lot of time — and we still do, for that matter — spreading the word, so to speak, talking to groups, organizations, doctors, and nurses, explaining the idea to them.

There was a lot of interest, but there was also some fear about the newness of it and there was some resistance to it. At the same time, there was also beginning to be a great deal of publicity on hospice. I think some of it gave hospice a sort of faddish appearance, which we did not want to encourage. We were very interested in the medical ideas of hospice — the idea of pain control and the idea of symptom control. That's what we really based our program on to start with. The problem was just the fact that people didn't know what it was.

There was also a problem — and there still is — in terms of any licensing or credentialing of any sort in Illinois. There still are no such things in Illinois, so there certainly weren't any then. We spent a lot of time with various agencies, (state agencies, regulatory agencies, and the Health Systems Agency in Chicago) trying to make them understand what this was and not getting very far. So we ran into this kind of red tape, which we found difficult. Finally, they didn't bother us anymore, because they didn't know what to do with us. I think they thought that we would just go away quietly, that hospice was something that was not going to last. Well, of course, that was a mistake, because it has.

R H   How did you get community support for your hospice?

A A   Well, we had open meetings in my living room every month. They were open to the community at large. Anyone who was interested in hospice could come. These meetings were very well attended. They still are. But we don't have them every month anymore, because we don't need to.

I would say that we got our major backing from the medical community to begin with — nurses, social workers, doctors. They were so happy to have a focus for their own energies as far as hospice was concerned that we received a lot of very quick support from them as well as a lot of ideas. We had requests to speak to various groups in various places. Getting support wasn't very hard to do. It's an idea that seems to appeal enormously to people. They're very interested in it.

R H Actually, the community support came quite easily.

A A Yes, I would say so.

R H There's no real resistance to it?

A A We used to think how well we were doing as far as this was concerned. You have to remember something, though, and that is that most of the groups we went to talk to already thought hospice was terrific. We weren't asked to go and talk to groups and organizations that were kind of leery of hospice. We were asked to go to talk to groups of nurses, groups of social workers — the kinds of people who would be interested in hospice. Our experiences were always positive, but we quickly realized that we were speaking to a certain segment of the population and that, perhaps, if we went further afield we might not meet with such acceptance.

R H How would you compare the initial reaction of the medical community with the reaction today?

A A I think the medical community, as a whole, is much more supportive, certainly more informed, and not as nervous about us as they were. I think they were somewhat nervous in the beginning that we were going to come in with a very critical attitude towards them, that we thought they hadn't done their job properly, and that we were the people who were going to do it for them. Some of this was true. And some of the initial interest we had from the public was because of a very negative attitude towards doctors and nurses on the part of the people who came to us.

I think we were also very fortunate in acquiring Doctor Michael Preador as our medical director, very early on — three years ago. Having a doctor as our medical director did a great deal to establish our credibility as far as pain control, as far as symptom control, and as far as this whole idea was concerned. Instead of being just a group of people who, perhaps, went and held hands — which is how I think some people thought of us in the beginning — we suddenly had new respect because of this doctor. Doctor Preador made enormous efforts with the medical community on our behalf, speaking, spreading the word, talking to medical groups.

We are very careful in our dealings with doctors. We want referrals from them. And we bend over backwards to let them know who we are and what we're doing. It's usually handled from doctor to doctor, which helps. Once they've seen that we are not out to steal their patients, that we are really there to work with them, if they want to stay involved with the patient, they are usually more accepting. That has helped us a great deal.

R H   Do you feel that the hospice movement has caused physicians to adopt hospice methods in the treatment of their own terminally ill patients?

A A   Of course we would hope that. But I don't think we have any hard evidence to back that up. And I don't know, at this point, of any way to gauge that. I think, perhaps, that physicians are becoming more aware of some pain control measures that they weren't aware of before. But then you know that good physicians have been practicing pain control for a long time.

R H   How is your organization funded?

A A   We're funded solely by private contributions, corporate contributions, and foundations. We are also fortunate enough to have quite a few memorial contributions from our families. We don't charge anything for our service. However, if the patient has Medicare, we do bill Medicare for doctor's visits.

R H   Are commercial insurance companies and Blue Cross billed?

A A   They are billed if they provide for home care, but only for the physician's visits. That's all. We are funded entirely privately.

R H   How does you program work?

A A   We have, at this point, 50 volunteers who work in teams of two. They go into the home once we have established that the case is a feasible one for us. Our doctor goes in first, with our nurse, to determine what physical problems there are, how we can be helpful, and how we can work with the physician on the case and with the existing home care agencies. We do not provide nursing care per se. We do work with the VNAs and with other local agencies.

When it has been established that the case is a feasible one, our volunteers go into the home and discuss with the family what needs to be done. They do anything that is necessary to help the family keep the patient at home. In other words, they may help cook, they may help clean, they may baby-sit. They may also do a lot of organizing of the various services that are available in the city. They coordinate these services. There are a lot of services available to help families. But if no one in the family knows about them or if the family is too tired and exhausted to make these arrangements themselves, we try to help. A lot of what volunteers do is simply provide support. They are available to the family on a 24-hour-a-day-basis. That is, they can be called day or night.

We have quite a few male volunteers who are enormously helpful. Sometimes we have male patients who are simply more comfortable with other men than they are with women. They can talk more easily to another man. If we think this is the case, we try very hard to put a man into the situation.

There is one thing, however, that we have to make sure that we do not do. We have to be sure, when we go into a home, that we do what the family wants us to do — not what we think we should do. Sometimes it is very hard, for example, for a volunteer not to get in and clean up a cluttered house or arrange things more conveniently in it. It takes a while for volunteers to realize that we can't do this. That's not what we're there for at all. If this is the way they live and if it is the way they want to live, it's not up to us to change it. Even so, there are some subtle kinds of things we can do when we want to get in there and tidy things up — either physically or emotionally.

I think it is very important for us to be totally family oriented, to be ready to carry out their wishes, and to give them — especially the patient — as much control over themselves and over their lives as possible during this period.

Scheduling is also important in our program. When does the family want the volunteers to come? During the morning? Afternoon? Evening? On weekends? After the two volunteers have made their initial visit together, they split and they don't go back to the home together.

R H   What are the qualifications of a good hospice worker?

A A   If I had to pick one, it would have to be a kind, compassionate, calm attitude — an attitude of caring. The caring attitude, I think, is one of the main strengths of the program. Sometimes it is the most helpful thing the volunteer can offer because these families have often been through a great deal of stress and strain by the time we come in — certainly a lot of hospitals, a lot of tests, and, sometimes, very unfortunate experiences. Sometimes just to listen is all we can do.

Another strength of the program is the fact that the volunteers have all kinds of backgrounds and they bring a kind of strength of their own to it. They bring to the program whatever their life experiences have been.

R H   What kind of orientation and training program do you have?

A A   We have a six-session training program for our volunteers. It's for anyone who wants to volunteer — whatever his background. It's a training session that we give as needed, usually twice a year. The prospective volunteers are screened and interviewed prior to being accepted.

What we try to do in this training course is to give volunteers a broad, fairly comprehensive background on hospice — on the idea, on the philosophy, and on the practical aspects — so that they will feel comfortable going into the home. Of course you can't cover everything in such a program, so we have continuing education sessions either once a month or once every other month.

We have a strong support system for our volunteers. Our

two volunteer coordinators are in touch with active volunteers every week about their cases and about what's going on. Our doctor is very accessible to the volunteers, as is our nurse, as is our executive director. We have other professionals who help us a lot. For example, we have a psychologist who is available to the volunteers at any time for discussing problems — problems they're having with the patient or problems they see within the family.

R H   Do you offer any pastoral care?

A A   We do. The vice-president of our board. Father Wilson Reed, an Episcopal minister, is very active. He's a volunteer himself. We have various other ministers and priests and a rabbi in the area who are available to us and to the volunteers.

R H   Do you have a burnout problem?

A A   I don't think we have had a lot of burnout per se. We have had volunteers who, for various reasons, have stopped volunteering. But I don't think it's necessarily been burnout. We take pretty good care of our volunteers. They have only one case at a time. They have a rest of at least a month, if possible, between cases. And they have time off for various things related to family and job. I don't think that we have a burnout problem. I believe there is a close feeling among these volunteers; they are readily available to each other. There is never a problem in having someone to talk to. There's always someone around.

As far as burnout in the family is concerned, one of the most valuable things we can do for a family is to stay with the patient for a few hours while the family gets out. Just to give them a break. We are also working on an inpatient unit so that the family can have a break. We can use it, among other things, as a respite — a place for the patient to go for a few days for pain control measures as well as to give the family a rest. Often there is a problem of physical exhaustion. It is very exhausting to take care of someone who is so very sick.

R H   It's a pretty heavy burden.

A A   For the family, yes. It's an enormous burden. And it helps

them if they can feel that we will back them up and that
we can take care of the patient so that family members can
pull themselves back together again.

R H   What have been some of the rewarding experiences that you
or your volunteers have had?

A A   People often ask me if this isn't depressing work. And,
actually, I don't feel that it's a bit depressing. I don't
think that any of us feel it's depressing. I think it's very sad
at times. We get into some very, very sad and difficult
situations, but the fact that we are doing something that
wouldn't be done otherwise is, in itself, very rewarding. The
attitudes of the families are fantastic. Most times, they are
very grateful, very appreciative. And because of the crisis
nature of this work, volunteers get to know the families
very quickly and are accepted into them very quickly. To
the kind of person that volunteers, this is very meaningful.

R H   Can you tell me about at least one rewarding experience
you personally have had?

A A   I have a patient right now whose family is one of the most
loving, close families that I have ever seen. Just being
around the family makes you feel good. This, of course, is
not always the case. This particular family has a lot of
money problems and a lot of other problems, too. Yet,
there is a kind of spirit, I guess you would say, that pre-
vails.

   The mother of the family is dying and she's fairly young
— 57 years old. Her best friend of many years has simply
moved in with the family to help take care of her. This
woman left her own family about a month ago. Of course
she goes home from time to time.

   Yesterday when I was out there visiting, the husband of
the family gave me a plant for Mother's Day. And, really,
I don't think that we have done that much for them, because they don't need a lot. They have each other. But
they are all so very frightened by the fact that the woman is
dying and by some of they symptoms and some of the
things she's gone through. So the volunteers provide a kind

of reassurance. I think we've been reassuring to them. It's such a pleasure, a joy to be around them. To see them getting through what is a terribly painful and sad experience, with this mother, wife, and friend. And yet, they manage. They have organized themselves to that. They are there, they are available, and they will do whatever they can to keep her as comfortable and as happy as she can be.

R H   You are saying that this has been an affirming experience and that it has kind of renewed your spirits?

A A   Oh, I think so. Very definitely. I think that the courage and imagination that our families have shown in so many instances of coping with really difficult situations is remarkable.

R H   Do you think the hospice can fit into the existing health care system?

A A   I think it is fitting in now — slowly but surely. It is certainly getting more and more recognition from the establishment. I think it is, yes.

R H   If there's anyone or anything in the establishment that sets up barriers to this kind of care, who or what would it be?

A A   It would probably be the mechanisms of the hospital. The hospice does not yet really fit into the hospital framework, because of all of the rules and regulations — the do's and the don'ts. We try to be much freer with our patients and our families than hospital staffs are. In addition, the hospital's effort to cure at all costs goes against our philosophy. Coping with everything that we would have to cope with in a hospital would cut down on our person-to-person approach.

    I think it's easier, in a way, for us to be independent and private. We don't have to cope with another board of directors and with a whole set of already established rules. We can do our own thing. Everyone involved with us understands the philosophy and is keyed into it. We don't have to continually fight battles with administration or with nursing or with any other departments that people in hospitals have to go through.

    On the other hand, we don't have the facilities of a

hospital. We don't have the backing of a hospital — the financial support, the public relations support, and that sort of thing. We've had to do these things on our own. Still, I personally think that I would rather stay independent because, philosophically, it is so much easier for us to get things done.

R H   What do you think about keeping a patient alive in the hospital as long as it is technically possible?

A A   If the patient is dying, if the medical profession has exhausted all of its resources, the place for the patient is not in a hospital. Hospitals are there to cure people. That's what they are *supposed* to be good at and that is what they *are* good at. Hospitals are not as attuned as they should be to the care of the terminally ill.

R H   I'm beginning to feel that doctors are finally being persuaded that it isn't necessary to keep people alive at all costs. I think in the last ten years there has been quite a shift towards the quality of care rather than the quantity of care. And I think the hospice movement has had a real effect.

A A   Good. I'm glad you do.

R H   It's been subtle, but it's gaining ground.

A A   I think, at present, there are some 800 hospices across the country in various stages of development. So this is something that is not just going to blow away. It is here to stay, whatever form it takes in the future.

R H   Will hospices ever be widely accepted?

A A   Yes. I think it will become more accepted. I think it is quite widely accepted now, actually. Once the medical community learns that the idea of hospice is solid, that we are not just a group of flaky people running around holding hands, that we can actually be useful to the medical community, the acceptance will come. It will come when the medical community sees that we are useful to them.

           Already, we get a lot of phone calls and a lot of referrals from visiting nurses and from social workers who don't know where else to turn. They are always grateful that there is a group that can come in and help them. Social workers, particularly, see us, more and more, as a useful organization, not just something to be put up with. Again, I think that when the doctors see that we do provide something for their patients that otherwise they wouldn't get, when they see that we do have their patient's best interest at heart, they'll come around. It's slow. It's really slow. But we can't be too impatient about it.

I've heard Doctor Cicely Saunders say that it took them seventeen years at St. Christopher's in England to really feel that they had established rapport with the local doctors. But this was really pioneering. Even so, seventeen years is a long time.

R H   And it takes patience.

A A   It sure does. You can't get impatient and you can't get irritated. The medical profession is a conservative group. And they always want to be sure about things. And I understand that. We have to prove ourselves. I think we have to prove ourselves in the area of high quality care. This is one of the areas that we in Horizon Hospice have been so concerned about — keeping Horizon small and doing what we set out to do in as excellent a manner as we can. We need to pay attention to detail — to the details of keeping the family together as well as to the details of the patient's medical care. These things often get overlooked in a big hospital or in a big nursing home.

R H   Where do you want to go from here?

A A   From here? I would like to see us have some inpatient facilities, preferably our own. Ideally, something that we would run. This is something we're looking into, but it's quite a way down the road.

It would be our own facility. It would be small and it would not be just for the terminally ill. It would also provide space for some nursing home kind of patients. One of the startling things that we have seen, from the very beginning in Chicago — and I'm sure it's true of any big city — is how many old, single people there are here.

We cannot take over the entire care or responsibility for their care, because there are so many people in this city who are lonely, sick, and alone — who don't want to leave their apartments. But when the time comes that they are too ill to take care of themselves, there is no alternative except to go into a nursing home. This they view with absolute dread. We have said from the beginning that we would like, in some way, to be able to do something for these single people who have no one. And I think this will be an adjunct to the inpatient facility.

R H   What else do you see down the road?

A A   I would very much like to see us on a firmer footing financially. I'd like to see us with some sort of an endowment fund. And I'd like to see us, perhaps, a little bit larger. We are up to between twelve to fifteen patients and families at one time. I think we could get up to twenty, but I don't think we ought to get much bigger than that. I'd like to see some kind of standards and criteria drawn up, probably by the National Hospice Organization. I think we should police ourselves, but there also needs to be some kind of accreditation — one that will do the job as far as quality control is concerned, but one that will not totally stifle the independent hospices. That's terribly important.

R H   Is there much dialogue among hospices?

A A   Oh, yes. I think that's one of the things that we feel very strongly about — helping other groups form. I think we were very helpful, for example, in helping the Meridian Hospice get started. Why should they go through some of the same things that we went through, if we can help them skip over it? I think hospice groups are full of very helpful people who are not necessarily possessive of their information. They are very willing to share.

Chapter 7

"SOMETHING FOR EVERYONE TO DO"

DIALOGUE WITH A VOLUNTEER COORDINATOR

After working for a brief period with a newly formed hospice in rural North Carolina, Lyn Fozzard returned to Chicago with a commitment. Her commitment first took the form of volunteer work with an already established hospice — the first one in the city. But that didn't seem to be enough for Lyn Fozzard. So when a colleague suggested that a hospice was needed to care for dying patients in their area of Chicago, she was ready, willing, and able to work hard to get the project off the ground. Now her commitmit takes the form of recruiting and selecting volunteers for the new Meridian Hospice. And she talks about it here.

E M   You are a registered nurse, aren't you?

L F   Yes.

E M   How did you get involved in hospice work?

L F   I think my interest began when I was nursing over at La-Rabida, which is a hospital for children. I was in the adolescent ward, where I was taking care of terminally ill adolescents. My initial introduction to the whole field of death and dying was through that experience and through Elisabeth Kubler-Ross, who came over to LaRabida to help us out.

     We have a farm in North Carolina in a very small mountain community. And a woman — from Chicago by the way — came down with her third husband and retired in Hendersonville. Her first two husbands had both died of cancer. So she felt a hospice was needed for our county. And she got enough people together and enough interest

81

E M   in it to get it going. So I acted as a consult during the time
      I was there.

E M   When was that?

L F   It started about four years ago. Then when I came back
      here, I inquired whether there were any hospices around.
      The only one I found was Horizon Hospice. And, lo and be-
      hold, the woman who founded it is married to a colleague
      of my husband at Billings Hospital. So I volunteered and
      worked there. I took the training course. Then I took a
      patient of theirs and worked with them until we got our
      own hospice started.

E M   How and when did you get it started?

L F   My office mate had been talking about how she felt our
      area needed something like this. So she and another friend
      and I invited Ada Addington to lunch to find out how to
      start one. And it was just like a pebble in a pond — the in-
      terest in the idea kept spreading and expanding.

      Our first organizational meeting, when we brought twelve
      interested people together, was held March 16 of 1981.
      We formed ourselves a board and we went on from there.
      Then less than one year later, with great fear and trepida-
      tion, we admitted our first patient. I had wanted to organize
      for at least three years. But we had some very eager, some
      very enthusiastic people who thought we were ready to take
      a patient last February — and we were.

      We now have a president, a vice-president and medical
      director, a secretary, two volunteer coordinators, and
      several committees, including a Community Affairs Com-
      mittee, a Bereavement Committee, and an Education
      Committee. We also have a team of fourteen volunteer
      doctors who make house calls and determine what things
      need to be done. All of us are volunteers. We have no paid
      staff.

E M   What happens if the patient has his own physician?

L F   It is understood, when a family calls us, that the hospice
      physician will be in charge of the team. And this is done
      with the cooperation and support of the patient's pri-
      mary physician. So far — and we have had eight patients —

it has worked very well.

Although all of our services are free, the family must contract with an appropriate agency for any skilled nursing care the patient might need. We do not provide nursing care.

E M   Where do your patients come from?

L F   They come from everywhere. They have been referred to us by social workers. They've been referred to us by physicians. They've been referred to us by people who have read about us in the paper. They come to us many ways.

E M   Your hospice is community-based, rather than hospital-based, isn't it?

L F   Yes. We are a community-based hospice that provides home care. We are, however, beginning now to do a survey of our neighborhood to find institutions that would be appropriate for us to ally ourselves with to get something that we think is very important — and that is respite care. In other words, when our patients become so ill that they can no longer be cared for in the home or when the family just needs a rest, the patient can come into the institution for a week or two.

E M   It's a backup.

L F   A backup, yes. Also, there are some families who really, desperately want to take care of their family member in their home. And then when they get home the patient deteriorates so much that they just can't do it. So we need a place like this.

E M   How much progress have you made in your search?

L M   Actually, no progress because we are just starting to go into institutions.

E M   What kind of reception have you had?

L M   Really very good. We have been contacted by a number of nursing homes who are interested in this kind of thing. But we have to be very, very careful about going into a for-profit institution to make sure that we have compatible goals.

If the legislation now being considered by the state legislature is passed, it will turn out to be a double-edged sword. We may then have "Kentucky Fried Hospices" all over the area.

E M   Have you given any thought to establishing your own respite care center?

L F   It would be prohibitive financially. We don't even have enough funds to support an office or a paid director, or any of those things.

What's more, we've been told that the freestanding hospices, even in England, are finding great difficulty staying afloat. And the ones in America are having trouble.

E M   You are one of two volunteer coordinators.

L F   Yes, our job is to recruit, select, train, and supervise volunteers.

E M   How do your volunteers come to you? The same way your patients do — through word of mouth?

L F   That's it. They are the people who stay around after one of our community presentations to ask more questions. We give them one of our brochures. And on the back of the brochure is a tear-off form for them to fill out and send in. A little later, we send them a letter than includes a volunteer job description. Then they come over for interviews with Sharon, the other coordinator, and me. And it goes from there.

In the first interview, we spend a lot of time on why these people want to do this, on what their past experiences have been — not only with death but with crisis — on what their coping mechanisms are, on what they do for distraction, on what they do for fun, on how much time they have to give us — things like that.

E M   What characteristics do you look for?

L F   A level of maturity and a real desire to commit themselves to this kind of service. People can be enthusiastic about many things without having a high level of commitment to them. You have to have a high level of commitment to this program. In fact, it takes commitment just to come in for an interview, much less try to find my office, which is in the basement over at Billings. Finding my office is a challenge in itself. If they've found it, you figure they're interested.

Originally, I would have assumed that most of the people who came to volunteer had some sort of intimate experience with the loss of a loved one. But a lot of them have not. And one of the reasons for their getting into this kind of work is to help them come to terms with death and to, in some way, prepare themselves for the loss of a loved one or for their own deaths. They admit this once we get around to talking about it.

E M   Is that a good reason for volunteering?

L F   Absolutely! Absolutely! In fact the people we ask to wait before becoming a volunteer are those who have suffered a great loss within the past year. It has been the experience of hospices who have been in the business much longer than we have that it takes a year, if not longer, for people to resolve their own feelings about this incredible experience. That is why we ask that they wait at least a year before they come into the program.

E M   Some people think that it's important for the person to have experienced a loss and other people don't think so. You obviously do not think it's a requirement.

L F   Absolutely not! But it's a big plus, because people who have gone through it are much more attuned to the kinds of things that can happen in families, and so forth. It's a big plus, but it's certainly not a requirement. In fact, we have two volunteers who are, themselves, terminally ill and who have been turned down by other hospices.

E M   Because of their conditions?

L F   Because of their conditions. Because the other hospices felt that these two volunteers would not be able to relate to the other patients or that they would be too intense. In interviewing these people, however, we found that they had an enormous amount to give and an enormous amount to share and that they were not going to unload their problems on the patients. If it came up in the course of conversation or if the volunteers felt it was appropriate, they would share with the patient that they, too, have a terminal illness. But they certainly were not going to go in and say,

"Hi, I'm dying too."

E M   What were their reasons for volunteering?

L F   They felt that they had a very special insight into the fears and the problems of someone who is terminally ill.

Now their terminality is not defined in the same way that we define it for the purpose of admitting patients. One of our criteria is that the patient have a prognosis of three to six months. These volunteers are certainly up and around and physically well enough to do it. Their deaths are not imminent. They are persons with various forms of leukemia and a prognosis of possibly two or three years. And this gives them a very special insight into what the patient is going through — one that none of the rest of us has.

E M   Next to maturity . . .

L F   And commitment.

E M   Next to maturity and commitment, what other things do you look for?

L F   A well-balanced and well-rounded life. We are immediately disturbed when someone says — after we've asked how much time they can give — "Oh, as much as you want." Anybody who is willing to come in and work full-time around the clock in this kind of thing worries us. It's pathologically unhealthy for them. We really like people with all kind of interests.

E M   What are some of the other things that you notice when interviewing someone?

L F   Oh, I'm trying to think. We have been very fortunate in the ones we've interviewed so far. I think we've suggested to only two or three that they would be more appropriate for some of our office work or some of our public relations work — something like that. In our talk they eventually have agreed that they were not quite ready to take on a patient or that maybe they never would be ready. But we need volunteers in everything, fund raising and everything else, so there are many, many areas that volunteers can work in. I was asked once, "How many volunteers have you rejected?" And I said, "Not one." There is something for absolutely everyone to do!

E M   What happens after the interview?

L F   They go through our training program. Once they have been through the program and have found that the hospice is really the kind of thing they can be comfortable with — and want to do — then we have them sign a contract. The contract simply spells out what their responsibilities are and what our responsibilities to them are — as far as supporting them, supervising them, keeping up a continuing source of in-service education, and those kinds of things. There is no time specified in the contract. We tell them, however, that we hope very much that they will stay with us a year.

E M   What do you expect of your volunteers?

L F   What do we expect of them? Their time. Many of them ask, "How much time am I expected to give? It has turned out — if you average over the whole spectrum of their association with the family — that the time averages out to be about three or four hours a week. Now there will be some weeks when all the family needs is a phone call. But we expect our volunteers to keep in regular touch.

E M   What else do you expect of your volunteers?

L F   Oh, there are other things. We expect them to attend our monthly patient care conferences. At those, the entire hospice team talks about the family and the patient and about how we can improve things. We also share experiences so that we can learn from each other.

E M   You said the entire team. When you say "team" who are you talking about?

L F   I'm talking about our medical director — who is the one who assigns the volunteer physicians — the volunteer physicians, Sharon and myself, the volunteers, of course, and then our consultants. We have volunteer consultants in the fields of psychology, social work, nutrition, physical thertherapy.

E M   How do you assign your volunteers?

L F   We always assign our volunteers two to a family, so that they are backups to each other. Not for that reason only, but also because we've found that, invariably, one volunteer has an immediate relationship — and a prolonged one — with the patient, while the other relates instantly to the family. And that has worked out very nicely.

There are really a lot of reasons why we do this. All of our volunteers, except for one, are working people who don't have vast amounts of time. We want them to be able to spell each other because of vacations and because of being out of town.

We spend a lot of time picking out the appropriate volunteers to go to the appropriate family, hoping that the chemistry and the time, and everything else, will match so that the end result will be that our volunteers will end up functioning like family members or very good neighbors or friends.

It's amazing to watch how the intensity of the relationship and the intensity of the experience have managed to cut a lot of barriers away. Relationships are formed almost instantly. For example, one of our patients was a 93-year-old man. We accepted him on a Thursday and he died the following Tuesday. Now that's not even a week. But in that space of time, our volunteers had become so close to his wife that when her husband died, she didn't want anyone else with her. She didn't want her family, she didn't want neighbors, she didn't want anyone with her except the volunteer that she had formed this extremely close relationship with. And it was Sandy who came and got the patient all ready for the funeral director, who kissed him goodby, and who stayed with his wife afterwards. This relationship has continued, even though they had known each other for five days. But this is the kind of thing that happens over and over again.

E M   Do you think there is any danger in such intensity?

L F   There could be. I'm sure you've read about burnout. But we're trying to protect against that — one, through our training sessions and two, through a psychiatrist associated with us who is a specialist in burnout. Then, of course, once a patient has died, we give the volunteer a rest. In other words, we don't assign the volunteer another patient the next day.

E M Is it true that the volunteer stays with the family for a period of a year afterwards?

L F Our bereavement team does. But it will depend entirely on how the volunteers are doing whether they stay on. We had felt initially that the volunteers — especially if the illness lasted over a long period of time and if the relationship became a very close one — would also be suffering loss and bereavement when the patient died. And they might not be the most helpful people for the family. However, if this has not happened and if the volunteers feel that they would be most useful to the family, they stay on. Staying on means that they call at specific intervals to see how things are going and to see what kind of help the family needs, which I assume will vary.

E M What support do you provide the volunteers?

L F Sharon and I keep in very close touch with our volunteers. And either Sharon or myself goes in with the medical director once we have gotten the referral. Then we keep that patient. In other words, our patients are divided between Sharon and myself. We keep in weekly touch with the volunteers to find out how things are going, to find out what areas they will need help in. They act as a kind of liaison between the family and the community. They know of services that the family may never even have thought were available to them.

When families run into problems in different areas, the volunteers come to either Sharon or me and say, "This family needs help finding a new home." Or "This family needs help getting a hospital bed." Or " This family's food stamps aren't coming through." Or "Is there some agency that can help get oxygen for this patient?" That's what we are there for.

If the volunteer runs into any kinds of problems or if he suddenly just can't take it any more, we step in as a backup.

E M Might it be that the volunteer couldn't deal with that situation but could deal with another?

L F   Oh yes.

E M   You wouldn't drop him as a volunteer?

L F   Oh good gracious no! There might be something in that particular situation that the volunteer just can't cope with any longer. And so we would try to find out what it is. This hasn't happened yet, but we anticipate that it could. We would try to find out what the problem was and then send in someone else who can meet the family's needs and assign the first volunteer somewhere else.

E M   What makes all of you so committed to the hospice?

L F   I think the spirit is reflected in a comment Cicely Saunders is reported to have made. It was to the effect that the only people who should be working in the hospice movement are those who cannot help but do so. In other words, those who, despite many personal and professional commitments, place the hospice goals at the top of their priorities are persons who are convinced that a comfortable and dignified ending of this life is a possibility for everyone desiring it.

Chapter 8

"A MEDICAL PROGRAM COMBINED WITH A SOCIAL PROGRAM"

DIALOGUES WITH A MEDICAL DIRECTOR AND A PROGRAM DIRECTOR

An early supporter of the hospice concept, Edwin Feldman, M.D., Medical Director at Chicago's Illinois Masonic Medical Center, worked hard several years ago to establish a hospice program at his hospital. Hospice Coordinator Kathleen Woods, ACSW, and her staff now work hard to maximize hope and enhance the quality of life for their hospice patients — those in the inpatient unit and those at home. In separate interviews, the hospital medical director and the hospice program director talk about the idea of hospice — about its potential, about its place in the system, and about its future.

E M   Do you have a special hospice unit or are your hospice patients spread throughout the hospital?

E F   Our hospice patients are not in the hospital as *hospice* patients. We have an oncology unit, which is for cancer patients, and patients in that unit may be potential hospice patients. That's one source of our hospice patient population. We also have outside referrals. The majority of these patients go home for care. The emphasis of the program is on home care. In some situations, however, the patient can't be cared for at home. Either there isn't enough support or the patient is too sick to be cared for at home. So we also have an inpatient hospice unit, which is located at Barr Pavilion. That's our skilled nursing facility, in which we've set aside four beds and a support area

91

for the family. That's our inpatient unit. Hospice patients come to the hospital only when they require intercurrent kinds of care that can't be dealt with at home or in the hospice unit. We try to avoid hospitalization as much as possible. But on occasion it is necessary.

E M   Are the four beds at Barr always filled?

E F   No. We sometimes will have two patients and sometimes we'll have a waiting list. One of our problems is the small-ness of the unit. We started out purposely with a small unit because we really were not entirely sure what the demand would be. Consequently, because there are only two two-bed rooms, it's difficult to mix and match — for instance, male and female — so we may have three patients and one empty bed because we can take only a male or a female. We may have four patients and a waiting list or we may have only two.

E M   How is the program organized?

E F   The program — and it is a program more than a place be-cause the inpatient unit is really a very small part — is managed by a team of people. That team of people is, in effect, an umbrella over the entire program. It oversees the patient regardless of where he is located — in the hos-pital, in his home, or in the hospice unit at Barr. That team consists of a medical director, a nurse coordinator, a hospice coordinator, a volunteer coordinator, a pastoral care coordinator, and the nurses who work at Barr Pavilion. They manage and have oversight control over all patients in the program. There is a plan for every hospice patient. And we supervise the provision of services for that plan.

If the patient goes home, we use the services of some of the local agencies — the VNA, for example. And then we add services that are not ordinarily given by these agencies— that is pastoral care, bereavement services. We also add some of the niceties of care that are provided by volunteers, such as running errands, sitting with people, helping clean house, cooking — all of the things that are not ordinarily medical problems. Volunteers, chaplains, social workers add on those services whether the patient is at home or whether he is at the Barr Pavilion.

E M   Are the rules and regulations at the Barr Pavilion the same or different than they are in other units?

E F   For hospice patients?

E M   Yes?

E F   They're different. They are different in this regard. Hospice patients are patients who are known to be dying. It is not expected that the patient can be cured. The chief thrust of the program is to make the patient physically, emotionally, and socially comfortable to the greatest degree possible. The nurses, the aides, and everyone else in that program know that their job is to make that patient comfortable, to keep him as active as is consistent with his condition, to keep him as in touch with his family and with the world as is possible, and to see to it that pain relief and emotional support is provided to whatever extent is possible.

We do as little testing as possible. We do as little of the usual hospital things as possible. We are not concerned with diagnostic procedures. We are not concerned with heroic therapeutic measures. We're concerned with relief and support and with involvement of the family, so as to keep people together as long as possible.

E M   Do you have more relaxed visiting hours?

E F   Yes. They're very relaxed. As a matter of fact, we have arrangements for families to come in and stay overnight. We would like to be able to extend that. We let kids come in. We let anybody from the family come in to the extent that they want to and to the extent that the patient wants them to. We encourage them. If they want to stay over they have their meals there. We have a little kitchen set up. They can make coffee and meals or snacks. They can eat together if they want to.

E M   Is the unit itself different from the regular units?

E F   The two rooms that the patients are in are not all that different, but there's a kind of family room with the kitchen. We don't really have as much room as we would like for family support.

E M   Are there any other differences?

E F   Well, only insofar as we can in a setting like that. This is
a skilled nursing facility. Even there we are constrained
by Board of Health regulations and by other kinds of regulations in how we can do things.

One of the problems of hospice is that it is a combination
of a medical program and a social program. To the extent
that it's medical, you have constraints relating to where you
put the hospice, to what rules you have to follow. To the
extent that it is a social program, other things have impact.
I would like very much to see the hospice in a setting
where there could be unlimited visiting, where the patient
could have an almost homelike setting, where the family
would come in and stay with the patient and eat with the
patient, where the pets could be brought in. I would like
to see a place that was as open as possible and as similar to
the patient's life-style as we could make it.

In England and in some other places, there are varieties
of settings. In some places the settings are essentially domi-
ciliary. It's an apartment building or a house. It's not a medical facility at all.

E M   Do you think a freestanding facility can make it in this
country?

E F   I don't think so. The experience seems to be that, at the
present time, hospices are about equally divided between
hospital-based and community-based. Experience is beginning to show that the hospital-based ones will probably
survive.

E M   And the community-based ones won't?

E F   I tend to think not. Not that that's good. I'm not prejudiced
one way or another. But so many of the services are not
medical, they are volunteer services — pastoral services, social work services, and program administration. They are
not services that are ordinarily funded by insurance companies, Medicare, etc. And because of that, you can't get
paid for the care. So the hospice has to be privately funded
or funded in some other way. Only insofar as the service

is medical can any portion of it be funded.

The problem comes when you recognize that the services are a combination of medical and social services and you realize that only insofar as they are medical can the services possibly be compensated. Therefore, I think hospital hospices are going to do better than nonhospital hospices. I think there's another reason, too. There has been some concern on the part of the government agencies and on the part of others about the potential for abuse of the hospice system, about entrepreneurally minded people coming in, taking — let's say — a nursing home, changing the sign over the door, and saying,"It's a hospice now." I suspect there will be some of that. So, on the basis of these things, I think it will be the hospital-based hospices that will survive.

The question really ought to be, "Will hospice programs survive at all?"

E M Do you think they will survive?

E F I think they'll survive, but I think it's iffy and I think there are some very serious problems involved, particularly in today's climate. We've found that there originally appeared to be a great groundswell of demand for this kind of care. People really wanted it. They wanted to "die with dignity." And I agree. I came into this at a personal level because of my own experience and I felt very strongly about it. I felt very strongly that we weren't doing the best job of dealing with people who were dying.

When we tried to approach the problem and deal with it, however, we found that it's costly, that no matter how efficiently you do it, there's a substantial cost. We also found that many people emotionally wanted to take care of their loved ones, but were not physically, emotionally, or geographically set up to do so. It's very hard. We don't live in big old houses anymore, where we can move around easily, where we're surrounded by members of the family who are there to help. People live in smaller houses or apartments. There's no extra room. And they don't have big families anymore to help out. It's often one person taking care of another and if it's a wife taking care of a husband, or vice versa, it's very hard. It's very hard to care for someone who is seriously ill and needs a great deal of attention and care. And no matter how much you're dedicated and how much you want to do it, there's a limit to what you can physically and emotionally do, even with the help of hospice volunteers and outside help. So we've found that there aren't that many people who can be cared for at home throughout the entire course of their illness. We did find, however, that we could deal with people longer at home than we could before. I think we made some impact there. But we also found that you have to have places for respite, if for nothing else. Every once in a while you have to give the family a chance to catch their breath or they couldn't make it themselves. It could tear a family apart emotionally.

We've also had trouble funding our program. There wasn't enough money available. We originally started out with a grant, which is now gone. It was never intended to be a permanent grant. If we charged people what it costs us to provide hospice services, most available funding would not cover it. When you include the cost of program administration, volunteer training, and so forth hospice care is fairly expensive to deliver. And lot of people couldn't afford it if we charged for these services. I have some real questions about what is going to happen in this economy about the hospice bills that are before Congress right now. If I had to guess at this time, I would guess that those bills will not go through.

E M   If they do, would they be a good or an evil or a mixed blessing?

E F   On balance, I think good. But the people who are doing it and the people who are paying for it had better understand what they are doing. They had better be clear about it. There is so much misunderstanding in this field that I suspect all kinds of conflicts and hostilities will arise. The funding agencies will probably be certain that the people who are providing services are doing too much, asking for too much money, abusing the system. And the people providing the services will be just as sure that the regulatory agencies are rigid, insensitive, and tightfisted. And to some degree, they're both going to be right. It's going to be tough.

I'd like to see it happen, but I hope that it is hospital-based, for one reason only. I think that, within the hospital community, we have the elements and some professional competences that, given the proper charge, we would be able to provide this care. We are open to review. We are open to audit control. So that if hospice care is going to be given, it probably ought to be given by hospitals. It ought to be clear, too, that a lot of the services will have to be volunteer services. We've got to go out and get people to do some of these things, because nobody ought to pay for those kinds of services. Who else is going to go out and do shopping? Who's going to stay with the patient so the family can get out of the house for a while? Who's going to do odd jobs? There are just a zillion things that most people take for granted that need to be done by volunteers. Not everybody can do all of the things that need to be done. It's one thing to shop for somebody, but it's another to sit with a dying patient who's vomiting, or worse, and deal with that. There are not too many people who can do this. It's our job to do it. Our volunteers and staff are trained to do it but the average individual is not.

E M Can and should all hospitals have hospice programs or units?

E F Oh, they probably can, but I don't think they should. I don't think there's that much hospice demand yet. I think we have overestimated the call. There was a time that people thought you should have a hospice on every block. That just isn't so. I think that, in the city of Chicago, ten hospice services would probably handle the present demand. This may change, of course, as more people become familiar with what it can do.

Right now, I don't think you'll find a big demand for hospice care, so I don't think every hospital ought to be doing it. I think there ought to be a few programs and there ought to be some economies of scale. As a matter of fact, we are probably going to start our own home health agency, hospital based, so that we can not only take care of our hospice patients but can also take care of others. This way we can staff more easily. It's hard to staff for ten patients or twenty patients. It's much easier to staff for fifty or seventy-five patients. So if every hospital had a little hospice program going, it would be economically inefficient.

E M   You think that hospice can fit into the system, but that it fits in best in a hospital-based program.

E F   I think it fits in best either in a hospital-based program or in a program that is closely affiliated with a hospital. I don't think that freestanding hospices — especially in the city — are the wave of the future.

* * * * *

E M   What are the criteria for admission to your inpatient unit?

K W   The three reasons for a patient to come into the hospice are for respite for the family (when the care at home becomes so overwhelming that the family needs a break), for symptom and pain control (which have to be carefully monitored), or for the last stages of the illness (when care at home is no longer possible or when the patient doesn't have the kind of supports at home that he needs).

Those are the three primary reasons for admission. In addition, the patient and his family must be aware of the diagnosis and the prognosis, even though they may choose to deny them. We have to know, at least, that they have been told. The patient and family must also consent to and want hospice care.

E M   Do you have any formal arrangement with the patient and his family?

K W   Yes. We do have a statement that they sign, which confirms that they understand the patient's condition and that they've been told about hospice care. The statement also describes what, essentially, will take place in the unit, in terms of physical care, nursing management, and symptom and pain control, and it points out that we will not do anything extraordinary to prolong life — like putting the patient on a respirator.

E M But you do give oxygen.

K W Oh yes. That's not considered to be extraordinary — oxygen, a nasal gastric tube, treatment for dehydration, and IVs, occasionally, are seen as comfort measures. We try to steer away from injections, if at all possible, because these people have been stuck with needles so much and another needle is not going to be very pleasant. That's why we emphasize oral medication, rather than injection. Pain can be controlled with oral medications, if taken regularly on a routine basis, rather than on an as-needed basis.

E M What's the most common reason for a patient to go into the inpatient unit?

K W I think it is because people are just not able to cope with a loved one dying at home, despite the fact that they may have agreed to the concept and, theoretically, want their loved one to die at home. It gets pretty scary at the end. Then there's the family's own emotional reactions to cope with as well as the physical care needs of the patient to deal with. It becomes very overwhelming.

E M How are you staffed down at the hospice inpatient unit?

K W We have four beds and our ratio is one nurse to four patients. Sometimes we have two nurses on one shift. But the full-time equivalents are 4.6. And that's really not enough. We need a higher ratio, I think. Perhaps not of staff, perhaps of volunteers.

Our program has difficulty getting daytime volunteers. Most of our volunteers, by nature of the area of the city we serve, are working people or students and they're busy during the day. Their availability for the program is evenings and weekends. We're actively recruiting daytime volunteers because many of the tasks that our present staff are doing could be done by volunteers.

E M I understand that the unit at Barr is more flexible in terms of visiting hours.

K W Yes, there are few restrictions on visiting hours. The other day we had someone come in at 10:00, with five children trailing behind her.

E M   At night?

K W   Yes, we don't always encourage that, but that happened to
      be when the woman was able to visit her aunt and she had
      her children with her. That was all right. We do allow a lot
      of flexibility as far as visiting, as far as staying, as far as stay-
      ing and sharing meals with the patient. Families are encour-
      aged to bring in foods, favorite foods for their loved one.
      The whole emphasis is to have the unit be as homelike as
      possible.

          The very atmosphere down there reflects an atmosphere
      or a milieu that says dying is a normal part of living. We do
      that by maximizing hope, which might seem paradoxical.

E M   How do you do that?

K W   The issue of hope, I think, is extremely important — an
      integral concept of hospice philosophy. When you lose
      hope, you lose your ability to function. Hope gets us go-
      ing. It gets us up in the morning and it gets us going out the
      door. I think we maximize hope by emphasizing the living
      of each day to the fullest, by maximizing the quality of life,
      and by helping patients and families to partialize hope into
      realistic considerations. Hope does not always have to be
      for cure. You see, that is usually what people equate with
      hope.

          This comes to me right now because I just had a long con-
      versation with the husband of a patient who has been ada-
      mantly opposed to hospice care because his concept of hos-
      pice was that it equals death and no hope. He cannot tol-
      erate that concept for himself or for his wife, even though
      she is dying and he can admit that she has less than a few
      months to live. It's the concept of no hope that some lay
      people have about hospice, which is very, very frightening.

          What I explained to the man was that we maximize and
      encourage hope, even though he and I both agree, perhaps,
      that hope is no longer for a cure. We can still hope for her
      to be able to return home. We can hope for her to get a
      bit stronger. We can hope that she has some days without
      pain. We can hope for her to see her grandchildren. There
      is always something to hold on to as far as hope is con-

67489

cerned. And this is not destroyed by the realism of the fact that this person's life is drawing to a close. We're helping them to deal with that. But we're helping them cope with it by emphasizing quality of life, not by preaching death and dying because that life is slipping away. Let's maximize what we have.

E M How do you do that?

K W I think by the normalcy of the environment. The hospice unit is not a sterile, cold place. The nurses wear regular street clothes. Families are encouraged, in fact strongly encouraged, to participate in hands-on care. The way we explain the unit is that we are there to help *them* care for their loved one. Oftentimes in a hospital setting the family has to leave the room when there are nursing procedures being done. At the hospice unit, rather than having the family leave the room when Mom has some physical needs the nurse is caring for, we encourage family members to stay, if they wish, for two days ago, Mom was, perhaps being cared for at home by her daughter who was giving her the bedpan and caring for her personal needs. The family is encouraged to stay in the room to participate — to help to bathe her, to comb her hair, to help to move her and to feed her. It's this kind of hands-on care that helps families and patients maintain intimacy and contact — physical contact — which is so important.

Participating in the care helps family members realize that Mom's arms are getting thinner, that she's developing a bed sore. The signs and symptoms of dying cannot be ignored. In that environment the signs of deterioration are acknowledged and the patient and family are able to deal with the situation realistically by talking about it. People are then more willing to talk about what's on their minds. You know, what their concerns are, what some of their fears are, and what some of their fantasies are about what might happen or about how the death is going to occur. The environment enhances and supports that type of dialogue with our staff and volunteers.

E M Do you prepare the family for the death?

K W   Yes, this is something that we do when appropriate. It's
      part of the anticipatory grief work we do with people —
      letting them know exactly what to expect. Then they're
      prepared for it, at least intellectually. It helps them to cope
      with the situation without a lot of panic. We'd like to do
      that with everyone, but not every patient and every fam-
      ily is open to that kind of thing. It really has to be done
      on a case-by-case basis.

E M   I understand that you don't have the unit always filled there
      at Barr.

K W   That's right. It isn't aways a hundred percent full because
      of several different factors. One is that people die and we
      may not immediately have someone on the waiting list.
      But oftentimes we have a waiting list far exceeding the avail-
      ability and people die on the waiting list, so to speak. The
      other thing is that sometimes people do not have the fi-
      nancial resources for hospice care.

         This is why we feel that the legislation before Congress
      is so important — the legislation on amending the Medicare
      act so that it will cover hospice care. If Medicare covers hos-
      pice care, we feel that private insurance companies will soon
      follow suit.

E M   Would Medicare coverage open the door for entrepreneurs
      to get in and take advantage of the system?

K W   Yes, there is that possibility, as we've seen with home health
      agencies and nursing homes. But all the more then do we
      need legislation that spells out what a hospice program is, as
      well as standards for care and measuring conformance to
      them. Otherwise — as someone so aptly put it — we're go-
      ing to have a string of Kentucky Fried Hospices.

         It's true that people, organizations, or entrepreneurs may
      set up what they call hospices, but not really deliver the
      kind of care that hospice, philosophically, is all about. That
      is a danger. But I don't think that that, in and of itself,
      should deter us from seeking reimbursement. With sufficient
      controls related to licensure, to effective standards, and to
      monitoring that care, it is hoped that reimbursement will
      come and that such reimbursement will be based on licen-
      sure.

E M   If I read Dr. Feldman right, he believes that the hospital-based program is really the only viable program.

K W   I think that, in the long run, he's reading the situation correctly. And I think I would agree with him. The hospital-based hospice programs have more supports that are already available and more resources at their disposal than the all-volunteer home-based programs.

E M   I understood from what Dr. Feldman was saying that he does not expect the hospice movement to grow as originally expected. Although there was a groundswell to begin with, it is his feeling that people are not now knocking down the doors of the hospices. Is that because a lot of people don't know what a hospice really is and how you go about getting hospice care? Is it partly that or is it that the idea will never be really accepted?

K W   Well, I guess I'm not as pessimistic as Dr. Feldman. The cultural basis of our society remains death denying and death defying. I believe that the lay community, as well as the professional community and the medical community, has not fully understood the concept. With any kind of program that deals with health care, you have to begin with physician education and attitude change. You really do. Look, for example, at how a physician feels when he is losing a patient to cancer or to any other terminal illness. The physician has strong feelings himself, whether or not he chooses to acknowledge them. Many times he cannot, or does not, choose to acknowledge those feelings. That influences, very definitely, his plan of care.

E M   What will it take, a generation of physicians, to get the idea of death accepted?

K W   Perhaps it will take that long before death comes out of the closet and is seen not as a failure in treatment but as a natural life event.

     The physician does not have to compromise any of his professional competencies in order to switch from the curing modalities to more concentrated caring modalities. I also think that the physician can provide what no other team member can provide. And that is the laying on the hands, so to speak, touching the patient, taking the pulse, or just any of the minor kinds of procedures that indicate to the patient and family that he is not abandoning them. That he will see them through this journey. That takes an awfully lot from a physician.

I was talking to a group of family physicians last week. We just sat around the table over lunch and talked about their experiences and about how they felt when they could do no more for a patient. We talked about the feelings of helplessness, and of impatience and of anger and of wanting to run away and of not knowing what to say. It just all spilled out. And it was so rewarding to me because *they* wanted to talk about it.

E M   Do you think that as long as they are trained to cure they're going to have those feelings?

K W   Yes, I do. I'm not saying to throw out the curative model. That works for many, many people. But medical education has to have elements of personal and professional sensitivity in it right from the very beginning. The physician does have to separate himself from the patient. That's understandable. He cannot be as competent in his diagnosis or treatment if he's not objective, but he also has to realize and understand the human aspect.

I'll never forget one young resident that I worked with at a large teaching and research hospital, part of the University of Chicago. His patient said one day that she was going to die. She felt very strange and she wanted to bring in her family from the South. Her blood gasses were fine. She didn't need oxygen, even though she insisted she have it. And so everyone thought, "Oh yes, she's just carrying on. She wants to bring her family up from Tennessee." So everyone just sort of passed off her sense of urgency.

The son came up and visited her and they made some plans. And that night about eight o'clock, I heard a code being called. I knew it was the patient's room number, so I ran up there. She had taken, as we say, the proverbial turn, in just a split second, and had died. They could not resuscitate her. She had died despite what the lab values had indicated. These young physicians were just going on the paperwork and had ignored the woman's sense of herself, her innate feeling that she would die soon.

That doctor was so angry and so upset. He tried to resuscitate her far beyond the point where it made any sense. It was obvious she was dead, but they would not give up. They tried this and they tried that. She was not going to budge. She had said her goodbyes and she had gone on her way. Well, the young doctor walked down to the conference room. He picked up the phone, threw it across the room, and said, "Dammit, she was not supposed to die. She was not supposed to die." He took it as a personal failure that this had happened to him. It was not so much that it was his fault, it was that he was personally affronted that she would do this to *him*.

On the other hand, I'm reminded of a situation that tells something about how we in hospice work are so convinced that we know about the proper way of dying. Dying can be peaceful. There can be lots of love and caring and sharing about the event between the patient and the members of the family. And I think we sometimes impose that model on our patients and families without having a real recognition of their own needs.

Last Sunday, a fourteen-year-old girl, who was a patient of ours, died. There's nothing like the death of a child to stir up feelings in caregivers as well as family members and friends. You can rationalize the death of an older person, but not the death of a child. There is no rhyme or reason to that existentially.

For some time, we had wanted Susan and her mother to be able to talk about the fact that she was dying. Every one of us saw that as being a goal. We tried to get them to do this. We talked to Susan's mother about this. She would ask the same questions — fifty times over of the nurse, the volunteer, the physician — "Should I tell Susan or shouldn't I tell Susan?" And she chose not to tell Susan that she was dying. Now Susan, I'm sure, knew. But Susan chose to deny too, to protect her mother. She kept talking about going to Florida and she knew she was never going to get to Florida.

What struck me so poignantly, when I went to visit the mother at the funeral home Monday, was that she had handled the situation in the way she was most comfortable with — in the way she had to do it. And all she had to hear from me Monday night was that it was okay and that she had done the best she could. That she had done it in the right way. Then she was able to acknowledge that "maybe I kept some secrets from Susan and maybe Susan kept some secrets from me."

It was then I realized once again that it was our needs that we were imposing on the family. We ourselves, had wanted to be more comfortable in dealing with the situation. We wanted it to be a good and appropriate death — *as we defined it* — because we had such feeling invested. But that was not the way the family had been able to define it for themselves. That experience brought home to me that it is often our own need that people do what we think is best. Sometimes they resist that and do what they need to do and that, in fact, becomes the best way of dying for them.

Chapter 9

"SIMPLY A CHANGE OF FOCUS"

DIALOGUE WITH A HOSPICE TEAM

Lutheran General Hospital is a large and progressive medical center in Park Ridge, Illinois. In 1981, it established a hospice program within its Home Care Department. One Friday morning over coffee, its dedicated hospice team — Coordinator Chris Koza, Pastor Leroy Joesten, Nurse Helen Main, Social Worker William Schack, Director of Volunteer Services Sandee Main, and Medical Director John Sage, M.D. — talked about their program. They talked about the hospital's commitment to it, about their own personal commitments to it, and about their volunteers' commitment to it.

L J   Lutheran General really has had a long-standing interest in care for the terminally ill. Back when Kubler-Ross was beginning her work, she came here for a couple of days of seminars — that must have been around 1970. She generated a great deal of interest and as a result of that particular workshop and the interest it generated, a special task force was set up. It was involved in trying to find ways in which we could better care for those who were terminally ill. One of the things that came out of the work of that task force was the development of a ministry to the terminally ill. It was established in the Pastoral Care Department. So it fell to that department to see what could be done further for these patients.

In 1973, I think it was, Doctor Ray Carey did a study in which several terminally ill patients were interviewed. They study was called "Living Until Death," and it was published in a number of journals. At about the same time, I accepted

107

a position here to develop a ministry to dying patients. A number of things came out of that. One was the Cancer Care Center that eventually developed in cooperation with a physician and a nurse. The center has been in existence for six or seven years. As a follow-up of this inpatient cancer unit, there came the desire of the hospital to complement it with some kind of program that would provide resources in the home. This was a direct follow-up on the hospice movement. It was in the middle seventies that the hospice movement was beginning to become popular around the country.

Lutheran General's hospice program, as such, has been open for a year, during which we have been caring for patients and families at home. It is strictly a home care program. We've had a general home care program at the hospital for the last eight years. And so it was natural that the hospice program, as a homebound service, be integrated into the home care program already in place.

The top administration of the hospital — the previous hospital president and the present hospital president — both have a very deep interest and strong support for any program of care for the dying. So the hospice program has had top administrative approval and support for as long as I have been here.

R H   Do you think that is essential for a successful program?

L J   Absolutely, absolutely.

R H   What would happen if you didn't get it?

L J   Well, I think it just wouldn't survive because of one very practical matter — money. Money is very hard to come by, at least at this point, for hospices. I think administrations must recognize that and claim hospice as a priority even though the institution may be struggling with financial restrictions.

C K   You need administrative support financially, but you also need administrative support in terms of recognition that the individual members of the team are involved in a special care program and, therefore, their responsibilities are going to be a little bit different than they would be on a general unit or in general home care. So, you need philosophical backing, too.

R H As well as material.

C K Yes.

R H How did each of you become involved in hospice care? Bill?

W S I was hired about a year-and-a-half ago, just as the program got started. At that time, I'd been working with an elderly population in the community, visiting older people in their homes. Over the course of about two or three years, some twenty of my clients had died. Most of them had died in hospitals. And their deaths had been very impersonal — for me as their counselor, for them, and for their families.

When I heard about a position opening up at Lutheran General in home care hospice, I was very interested. I was interested in working with people at home as well as with people who were terminal. So I interviewed for the job and got it. That's how I got into hospice work.

H M I had been taking care of terminally ill patients at home, on my own, for about six or seven years. But I didn't have the availability of any kind of support system, which I just felt was a necessity. Then, when I heard that there was going to be a hospice program here, I became rather persistent about wanting to be interviewed for the job.

E M Were you a staff nurse or were you caring for patients all on your own?

H M I was doing it on my own, but I was also doing it for some agencies. I had come from an intensive care setting to home care. And I realized that this was the kind of work I wanted to do.

R H How long have you been here?

H M Since January of last year.

R H Chris?

C K I'd been working with cancer patients for about seven-and-one-half years. I'm a registered nurse. I'm serving here both in a nursing capacity, caring for a caseload of patients, and as coordinator of the program. Prior to coming here, though, I had worked with cancer patients in an acute-care setting. When you are dealing with cancer patients in an acute-care setting, you are dealing with a gamut of emotions, as well as a gamut of stages of the disease.

I think that experience made me more acutely aware of the lack of options available to patients and their families. It also made me aware of the additional support they need in a hospital setting, but even more so of the additional support that would be necessary to make it possible for the patient to die at home.

R H   Doctor Sage, how did you become the medical director?

J S   I got involved because I was in private practice. And in my practice I was helping families keep their dying loved ones at home. In doing this, I had an opportunity to see that hospice worked, that it was effective, and that it was good for more than just the patient. I also saw patients in the hospital — patients who needed care, but probably did not need to be in an acute-care hospital. So when Lee Joesten asked me to come to a meeting of the Task Force Planning Committee, I came very willingly.

S M   I became involved because I am director of volunteer services at the hospital. As such, I am responsible for any volunteer activity that is done on behalf of the hospital. So, because the hospice does use volunteers, this is a piece of my job.

R H   In America, we have been a little reluctant to become involved with pain control methods that have become popular, particularly in England, because the patient may become addicted to drugs. How do you feel about this?

J S   I thought, when I became involved in the hospice program, that this would be an incredibly large problem — a problem that we would have a great deal of difficulty in controlling. And sometimes it is. But I think by and far (and we've talked about this in some of our discussions) that there have been other symptoms and discomforts that have caused more problems than pain per se.

The experience of others — those who have had more experience than we have — has been that pain really is not such a large problem. The Brompton cocktail per se is not being used so much here. We quite frequently recommend a variation of it that is just an oral morphine solution. The problems of addiction sometimes do occur, but we have not seen it. The family worries about that. Sometimes you see physicians who still have this concern about the dying patient being addicted — as if that were something so bad.

I think we are all becoming more confident. We tell people that we can really control their pain. Many times there are side effects — nausea, drowsiness, things like that. Many of these side effects from the pain or from the morphine solution can be controlled. Again, in our experience pain has not that often been a recurring, predominant problem.

R H   What are some of the problems other than pain?

J S   We have most recently been involved with people who have had bowel obstructions, vomiting — things like that. It's really very difficult for the family to observe and for the patient to have recurring problems like these.

R H   What about euthanasia?

J S   In looking at what our experience has been with our forty-five patients, I would say that, certainly, there have been people who have wanted to die.

H M   We have had several who asked their spouses to do away with them during the course of their illness.

R H   Was this as the result of pain or of the awareness that they were going to die?

H M   In the most recent case, the patient was really living longer than we expected. And he was worried that he was a burden on his wife — the day in and day out care. His concern was probably also worrying the spouse.

C K   I think that the response Doctor Cicely Saunders would give — the one she gave on the CBS program *60 Minutes* — is that the hospice should be one of the movements that make euthanasia an unnecessary entity because, hopefully, with all of our resources we can deal effectively with the patient's needs — the physical needs, the pain, the bowel obstruction, the spiritual needs, the psychological needs, the suffering.

E M   Do you think that's realistic?

C K   I think for the great majority of people, yes. Certainly, there will be some whose needs are just a little bit deeper and who will require additional support. Hospice will never promise that 100 percent of the patients will not feel pain, but we will certainly work hard and put all of our efforts together so that the greatest amount of comfortableness possible is provided and maintained for the patient and for the family. The family is just as much our concern as the patient.

J S   Over the last year or so, I don't think that we ever came to the conclusion that euthanasia would have been a necessary or even a desirable alternative.

L J   I like the way that Cicely Saunders and St. Christopher's Hospice talk about euthanasia, about the understanding of the word. *Euthanasia* in my recollection implies a good death. And that does not mean mercy killing. It means a good death.

       And I think hospice represents efforts to make dying bearable. And even more than that — to help people find, within their dying, meaning and purpose and some kind of direction. And that is very difficult. I think that the kind of people who may not be satisfied with hospice are the people who may be strongly independent, who are not really open to that kind of quest anyway, who are gradually coming to a greater and greater dependent state, and who finding themselves in that state find life totally unbearable. So, they elect to take their own lives or to plead for someone else to take it.

       I don't think that the statements "I would like to die," "I would like to get it over with," are all that unusual. I think a lot of people either think that or say that at one time or another. Those who would actually, if they were given a chance, accept someone's offer to take their lives would probably number very few. I think it's a natural, though, a natural wish in the state of suffering — and not just physical suffering, but also spiritual suffering and emotional suffering, suffering from being a burden — for people to want their lives to end.

H M I recall one patient, just recently, who asked his wife to get rid of him. He didn't say in what way or anything. As it turned out he lived longer than expected, but had a very decent and pain-free last two weeks. In fact, he had all of . his family at his house for Easter Sunday. Then, even though he was terribly weak, he played Scrabble® one day. The man also went outside two times to look at his house — front and back — to see the flowers that were coming up. Prior to that time, he didn't want to live. His wife was exhausted, but I think that those last few days will be a real comfort to her — knowing that he did enjoy some time. No matter how little the time, there was some quality and value to it in those last few days.

R H Would you tell us more about the volunteer aspects of your program?

S M We have five volunteers who have been with us for this year. And we are now in the midst of another training program in which we have fifteen prospective volunteers who are going through a thirteen-hour program. We have found, and I am sure Helen (nurse) has found, the volunteers especially supportive to the team. They are available during the week to do many kinds of things with the patients or with their families. They have worked with the blender and made food more edible for the patient. If there are small children in the home, they take them to the park or transport them to nursery school if that's a need. They visit with the patient and act as a support system for the family member. They give whatever kind of assistance and support they can to the family. During the bereavement period, the volunteers have been very, very active. I think the whole team would agree that it wouldn't be a total program without volunteers.

R H What do you consider the qualifications for an effective volunteer?

S M I think the first one, probably, is a love of people. Someone who meets others easily. I think they also have to be genuine in forming relationships and in really caring about people.

R H   How much time a week do volunteers usually give?

S M   It varies. It's not the kind of job in which you can say, "We'll need you every Tuesday from two to four," as we do with traditional volunteers. When needs arise within the family, volunteers need to and want to go there. Some weeks, it might be six hours or it might be an hour on the phone every day or it might be a chunk of two hours. It varies so.

R H   Is there a dearth or a plethora of people who want to volunteer?

S M   The first time we recruited, an article went into the newspaper. I believe we had about ninety responses over a two-week period. At the time, we had set a goal of selecting twenty who would meet our basic criteria.

R H   Which you enumerated.

S M   Yes, but in addition, we also think that the person should have experienced some kind of loss. As they begin to talk about that loss during the interview, a judgement is being made — by the hospice director or by the pastor or by the social worker — as to how well that person has handled that loss. If they appear to have handled it well, and if they really want to help other people, they are selected. Now this last time, we went through very much the same process but response was not as great. Even so, we were able to select from, I would say, twenty-five people. We selected sixteen.

One of the other criteria is that the volunteer attend all four training sessions. So even though a volunteer is very interested but can't attend one of those sessions, he eliminates himself.

E M   What reasons do volunteers give for wanting to do it?

C K   It runs the gamut. Some, as Sandee indicated, have experienced a death in the family and feel the need for some additional support. We have, I think, three or four nurses in the program right now who, because of their own clinical practices, understand the hospice concept and realize the need for the additional support in the home. Although these nurses do not act as nurses in the program, they, perhaps, have a greater degree of comfort in dealing with some of the physical aspects of the illnesses. They have a commitment to it from that aspect. Others are, frankly, just common, everyday kinds of friendly neighbor people who have heard about the hospice concept and want to reach out to people and families who might need their services.

R H Do you think your volunteers should be trained even beyond your basic thirteen-hour program?

C K When Lee and I spoke about it last week, one of the things we talked about was the fact that we are not training grief counselors, we are not training psychotherapists. We've screened the volunteers as closely as we can to be certain that there is not an underlying agenda related to meeting their own personal needs.

I think the most important thing is what Sandee brought up — the fact that these volunteers really are very caring individuals who are willing and eager to give of themselves and of their time to patients and their families.

S M That thirteen hours doesn't represent the only information and training they get. We did have some in-service sessions on listening skills and on signs and symptoms of impending death. And we have more things planned. We are going to give them more information as they go along.

I think one of the most important things is one we haven't discussed yet. We have a monthly support group meeting for the volunteers. One afternoon a month, all the volunteers get together with members of the hospice team and discuss the issues or concerns they have in dealing with any particular patient. They share that with hospice team members and they share it with each other. It's been, I think, a very valuable experience, because we can very specifically address what's happening with particular patients. And they're all learning from it. In the future they may run into situations that are very similar and will benefit from knowing how it was handled by another volunteer or from the responses they received from the team members.

We also have team meetings Monday and Friday. And there have been times that we have invited the volunteers.

When a particular patient has some presenting problems that could benefit from the group approach or when we're concerned about a specific issue, we invite them. And we feel that the volunteers have a lot of input to give us and, in those instances, we invite them to come to our meetings.

R H   Can your program function without volunteers?

W S   No.

S M   We have some families that can function without volunteers, but our total program could not function without them.

R H   How closely do you identify with the patient and how do you feel about that identification?

W S   I think that I have probably learned a great deal from the contact, however close it was, with patients and their family members. I have been surprised sometimes to find that there aren't always answers to give patients or to family members. I've also found that, somehow, people have a way of explaining or accepting their own deaths. And it's very different for everybody. Some people can never really accept termination of life. Some people just can't come to terms with it so that they can either talk about it or experience a sense of comfort.

But I would say that most people, at least, have been able to feel comfortable with it. I have sort of been nourished by the patients and the families' sense of comfort. I think it's really a give and take. You also never know when you're really going to be able to be most helpful. It changes with different situations.

R H   Do you ever cry when your patient or client dies?

W S   No, I haven't cried about the deaths of our patients.

R H   How do you think you would feel if you did find yourself crying or suddenly breaking down?

W S   Oh, I would feel good. I would feel good about it. I don't think I would feel needlessly anxious or concerned that this was inappropriate or excessively emotional on my part, because I'm sure that the piece of me that I am able to give people is, perhaps, the best thing I'm able to give.

C K   I think that people involved in hospice certainly do experience the grief process, but not to the same extent that the family might. It depends on the intensity of the involvement with the patient and with the family, as well as the length of the involvement. Certainly there have been tears shed.

R H   You've shed tears, Chris?

C K   Over the many years of working with terminally ill patients, oh, most certainly. I think that what's a bit different with hospice is that when we begin to work with the patient we do know that he has a very limited life expectancy. So, in some ways, we are more prepared for what is going to happen. That doesn't mean that we still don't cry with the patient about some happy or sad memories of the past, as well as about some unfinished business that will never be finished.

R H   So you don't think it's unprofessional to break down and shed tears.

C K   I don't think they even teach that in nursing school any more.

W S   I haven't cried about the loss of any of our hospice patients, but I have cried about the death of three or four patients that I'd worked with before I came here. And as I think back to why I cried in those situations, I found it was because these were very lonely deaths. I felt very bad, very sad, and, perhaps a little depressed about how lonely these people were when they died. I have not felt that about our hospice patients. Our hospice patients have not been lonely when they died.

H M   I get close to most of my patients. Some of them I haven't been involved with very long when they've died or, for some reason we have not had that closeness that I have had with other patients. In some cases, I think they rely on me too much and then I get too involved with them. I'm saddened, sometimes, that I didn't know these patients when they were well. That I'd never known them before. Sometimes I've cried because I'm relieved that they've died. I think, in some instances, it's been too much of a struggle for them.

J S   Since I've been distant from these patients, in the sense that they have their own doctors, I have not shed any tears that I can recall. Over the past couple of years, I have cried over some of my own patients, primarily because they haven't died on my schedule. There were things that I was hoping to discuss, to bring up, to share with them about their impending death. They died before I was ready. And that was real painful.

R H   Beautiful. Do you feel that the medical profession — I'm speaking of doctors — is becoming more humanized in the sense that it's okay for a patient to die. That it isn't something horrible.

J S   I'm told that fifteen years ago, when I wasn't practicing medicine, doctors' attitudes toward discussing death was different than it is now. This is information that doctors thought patients didn't want to know. Now, if you took a poll of doctors, 90 percent of them would probably agree that their patients do have a right and a need to know about their diagnoses. My impression is that now doctors are discussing death with their patients and expressing their own feelings much more freely. I think they are more comfortable with the fact that their patients die.

E M   How do you explain the actions of physicians who appear to avoid the patient in the last stage of terminal illness?

H M   It's the feeling that patients and families frequently have of abandonment. Physicians are not making house calls and patients are not going to offices. They are seeing us and we become intensely involved.

C K   That physician has provided an important continuum of care in that he did recommend the hospice team.

E M   Is there ever any room for joy or humor in hospice work?

C K   Of course. Hospice is about living. It's helping the patient to live until he dies. My goodness, I think that 99 percent of what we do is help to establish a quality of life — to make possible things like going around the house, looking at the front and back, and talking about where the flowers should be planted.

H M   People can be funny about their deaths, too. I am thinking about one patient we have whose neighbor died recently. The two couples have cemetery plots that are adjacent. And our patient wants to be sure that she's not buried next to the husband of the lady across the street because she doesn't want him to reach over and touch her.

She can say this kiddingly to us now, even knowing that her death is going to be a reality soon. It came out in a very serious conversation that we had when we told her that the woman across the street had died. Her neighbor's death was very hard for her to accept because she knew that she was probably next in line.

L J   We were able to enjoy that remark with her. And she knew that she could say it because she trusted that we could appreciate the humor in that. A person's limited life expectancy does not negate the opportunity to laugh.

H M   One of the things that Joy Ufema asks when she interviews a volunteer is "What is your favorite joke?"

R H   What is your relationship with the hospital's medical and nursing staffs?

C K   One of our ongoing efforts is to help everyone involved to be as comfortable as we are with hospice care being just a continuation of the patient's care. It's not "this is the end of the line. There's nothing else I can do." It's simply a change of focus.

R H   Then you aren't resented?

J S   The only friction that I was ever aware of as a member of the team was that the physicians and nurses wanted to make damned sure that we were qualified to get involved. They wanted to know what our credentials were. They wanted to know who we were. There was no dumping syndrome. There was no "Let them take care of him now." It was "Hey, are you going to care for him as much as we care for him?" I have a feeling now that everyone is very happy that the hospice is here. I think it helps them to feel better about what they do.

Chapter 10

"BEING A FRIEND IN NEED"

DIALOGUE WITH A NEW VOLUNTEER

In June of 1978, volunteer Randolph Hughes retired after thirty-one years as a medical technologist at Billings Hospital in Chicago. But retirement for Randolph Hughes did not mean burning his bridges with medicine or with Billings. He still goes back to the hospital's laboratory one or two days a month to help out and to keep his hand in. Since December of 1981, he has also been a volunteer at the Hyde Park-based Meridian Hospice. Having completed his training, he is now awaiting his first assignment. He talks here about his motiviation, his involvement, and his commitment to hospice.

E M How did you happen to become a hospice volunteer?

R H My first knowledge of hospice care was in Los Angeles. I had a sister who had cancer. And when she got to the terminal stage, the hospice came in and helped take care of her. (I think the hospice was located in Anaheim — somewhere near Los Angeles.)

The hospice people were just wonderful with her. They brought in all the supplies. They brought the medication and they explained the medication to us. They provided the various equipment and supplies she needed — beds, wheelchairs, toilet things — all the things we needed. They also gave us information, so that we would be prepared for what was going to happen. Hospice volunteers came almost as quickly as a policeman could when you called for help. And sometimes they came out just to sit with her. I was really amazed that they would do this. There was no charge or fee or anything.

E M   How did your sister come to have hospice care?

R H   It was probably through the hospital — Daniel Freeman, a
       Catholic hospital there in Los Angeles. She had gone there
       all during her illness, so they had probably asked if she
       would like the assistance of the hospice group, once they
       had given up on her.

E M   Did your sister have family out there?

R H   Only her husband. Over the two-year period that she was
       ill, I made about five or six trips out there.

E M   How did her husband feel about the hospice?

R H   He was very, very impressed with it. He thought it was the
       greatest thing because of the kindness of the people — not
       only in what they were doing, but in the manner in which
       they did it. I suppose you would say they were just good
       human beings.
           My sister was in and out of the hospital. In fact she was
       in the hospital about four days before she died. My brother-
       in-law never quite accepted the fact that she was terminal.
       As a result, whenever she was in severe pain he would call
       the hospital and I feel, sometimes, that out of sympathy
       for him, they would take her in the hospital for a few days.
       The last time, they kept her until she began to have what
       is called a death rattle. Then we brought her home.

E M   Were any members of the hospice team with her when she
       died?

R H   No. They had been there that day, but she died at nine
       o'clock at night. Both my brother-in-law and I were there
       and we were both taking care of her. We knew what to
       expect.

E M   How long did she have hospice care?

R H   I imagine about two months. I wasn't there. I got there
       just at the end. I was very impressed with the hospice, nat-
       urally, but I didn't know that there was a hospice in ex-
       istence in Chicago.

E M   When did your sister die?

R H   It was about a year-and-a-half ago. She died in February
       of 1980. When I came home, I brought her body with me.
       And when anybody wanted to buy flowers, I took the

money instead and sent it to the hospice in California. And
to people here who wanted to make a contribution, I
suggested making it to the hospice.

E M   If you didn't know that hospices existed in Chicago, how
did you get involved with Meridian?

R H   Last December at a Christmas party, when Dr. Bernard
Levin and I were in a conversation, he mentioned his part
in organizing the hospice in Hyde Park. I then simply said
to him, "Why is it you have never asked me to help out
with some of these things, which I have time to do?"

He didn't even answer me. He got up and went over to
where Betty Wissler was. In the next second she was right
beside me saying, "We would love to have you in our
group. We have a training program going on now." So that's
how I got involved with hospice here in Chicago. Afterwards she told me that there was a hospice on the north
side.

E M   But you preferred to go to the south side.

R H   Well, I had already committed myself because I didn't
know the existence of the one up here.

E M   What made you want to get involved with the new hospice?

R H   My mother and father have both died, my four sisters and
my two brothers have died, and I've helped take care of
every one of them. I feel I have practice in doing this. I
can't say that I really enjoy this, because it's not something
one enjoys. But knowing that you are doing something to
help someone is important. I know that, in all of the times
that we've gone through having someone in the family die,
it's a very, very trying kind of time. I just feel that if I can
help somebody else, I'm willing to do it.

When my father died, my mother — in her grief — said
"Who is going to take care of me?" And I said, "I will."
And at that very moment, I said kind of a prayer. "Let
me be the one to take care of them all." One of my sisters and I were in California when our sister there was going to have surgery. The morning she went up for surgery, I was so broken up about the whole thing. I remembered that prayer and thought "I asked for this." I had never

told anyone about that prayer. And I didn't know what it was going to involve. I was grieving and I was going to have to suffer to take care of her. I was very, very despondent at the time.

E M   Were members of your family ill over long periods of time?

R H   Not all of them. My mother's illness was not very long. My father's was only about 12 days. He had a massive stroke. One brother had rheumatic heart disease and ended up having bacterial endocarditis. He was 42 years old, I believe, when he died. He had to have an amputation and had other complications. Another sister had a two-year battle with cancer. And my oldest sister, who had hypertension, had many strokes before she finally died. I had another brother who died of pneumonia and various complications. And then one sister had bypass surgery. My sister who died in February never knew that our other sister had died on New Year's Eve.

E M   You were a very close family, weren't you?

R H   Oh yes, every one of us.

E M   When you were taking care of members of your family, was it a psychological need, a practical need, or both?

R H   It was a combination of both.

E M   It takes a lot of strength to deal with the kind of losses you have had to deal with.

R H   I'm beginning to feel a little different about it now, but it took a long time.

E M   Were you a religious family or did you get your strength from each other?

R H   We were a religious family. My mother was Methodist and when we were kids we all went to church with her and to Sunday School. When it came to joining the church, she said, "I would like to have you wait until you know what faith you want to accept. And when you do it, do it with your whole heart and soul." With that remark, she got two Catholics in the family. I think the major thing for her was that we accept religion.

E M   I would imagine that your faith provided you with some of your strength and some of your coping mechanisms throughout all of this.

R H   Yes, you do draw on that. I have often wondered how an atheist or an agnostic feels when he is in the depth of despondency. I wonder what he has to draw on.

E M   So you were prepared for hospice work — both the physical and the emotional strains — by your life experiences?

R H   Yes.

E M   What happened after you indicated your interest in the hospice?

R H   Then I took the usual course of lectures.

E M   How long was the course and what did it include?

R H   I think it was eighteen hours, and it consisted of lectures by professional people.

E M   Were most of the lecturers from the University of Chicago?

R H   Some of them were people who are in the hospice — doctors, nurses, dieticians — most of them work there in the University or are associated with the University of Chicago Hospitals.

E M   What were some of the specific things that were included in your training?

R H   We were trained to do body rubs and things like that. We had a physiotherapist speak to us. Then after the demonstrations, we practiced on each other the various things one does to make a patient more comfortable in bed — body massage, foot massage, elevation of the feet, various things of this sort. Whatever is needed in terms of the ailment. Positioning the patient in bed so that he doesn't get bed sores. Positioning patients is very important for those who can't get out of bed. We learned various other things that you can do to keep patients from getting body sores or ankle sores from the friction of the sheets. We learned the importance of getting patients out of bed, if at all possible, and into a sitting position.

Another thing I learned is that it is so important to let the patient make his own decisions as long as he is capable of doing it. It is very important to allow them to make decisions about how they want to be turned and about other things they want. In that way, they feel they are still kind of in command of themselves, that they can ask for things to be done for them and have them done.

In the hospice class, I also learned that medication can alter a patient's sense of taste. That was something I was not aware of. When my sister was sick, she would think she wanted a certain food and then reject it when it was offered. At the time, we were very insistent that, since she had asked for it, she should eat it. Now I think I was being a little unkind by being insistent that she eat things that she didn't want. But in my innocence or lack of knowledge, I didn't know that medication could change the taste of food.

We were also told in our lectures that we must respect the individual — whatever his religious denomination. We are there not to judge; we are there to help that person.

E M   What do you think it takes to be a good hospice worker?

R H   To be a good hospice worker, I think you have to have had experience with death. Someone has said, you can't make the statement, "I know how you feel." I don't ever think I would make that kind of statement. You really don't know how they feel; you only know how you felt at the time you went through it. If someone comes along and puts his arm around you and embraces you, that does more than any words he could have said. You knew he was with you. Sometimes that's all the communication that's needed. When you're caring for a patient, I think mother wit is also required.

E M   Mother wit? I've never heard of that before.

R H   Yes. Well that's something you inherit.

When we're caring for patients, we leave ourselves open for whatever the family wants us to do. If it's going to the grocery store or if it's sitting with the patient while the family member goes out, fine. Anyone who has been exposed to illness as much as I have has had to do these kinds of things for family or friends.

E M   What kind of emotional support do you think you will need to be able to cope with continuing relationships with dying persons?

R H   I don't think it will depress me too much. I cannot say that
       I can do it with the same feeling that I did with members
       of my family. I think I can do it very well and not have it
       affect me too much.

       The fact that I am helping someone in the hour that
       they really need it helps make up for the sad part of it.
       And I'm looking forward to being of help to that person
       rather than thinking of my own feelings.

E M   How long do you think you will stay in hospice work?

R H   For some time. One thing that helps me out greatly is my
       own personal philosophy. I am a person who, at the end
       of the day, asks, "What have I contributed today?" If it
       comes out zero, I feel kind of bad. I also feel now that I'm
       retired, there will be a lot of days that I will do things self-
       ishly — just for my own pleasure. And I don't think that's
       contributing a heck of a lot to suffering humanity.

E M   You'd like a better balance at the end of the day.

R H   Yes, but I expect that hospice work will make up for a lot
       of that. If I do something worthwhile during the day with
       the patient, then I can go to bed with a free conscience.
       And at the end of the week I can feel that I have contrib-
       uted something in those seven days.

E M   You have completed your training and are waiting to be
       assigned to a patient, isn't that right?

R H   Yes. I was waiting one whole weekend for a patient. Our
       coordinator called and asked if I would take the patient
       and I said yes. Afterwards she called and said the man had
       been in a very, very depressed state for a long time. He had
       changed his mind after agreeing to hospice care.

       But just because I don't have a patient doesn't mean
       that I'm not available to help in another way. Being with
       a patient is not the whole story. There are a lot of duties
       to be done to keep an organization like this going. I'm
       willing to lick envelopes to get the hospice on its way. If
       I had a patient, I would spend maybe eight or ten hours
       a week with him. I can just as easily spend those eight
       to ten hours doing something else.

E M   Do you think the hospice movement will grow?

R H   There are some people who predict that hospices won't last, can't last. But there are people who are going to volunteer to do these things. And once a person has been a recipient of hospice care, the word will get around. I think the problem is to make the general public aware that hospice exists, which Meridian is doing. Representatives are going around to various churches to make them aware of the hospice. Another volunteer and I visited the police station last week to alert the police to the fact that we exist, so that if we ever need their help or their protection, they will know who we are. I think it will spread and that when hospitals have terminally ill patients they will make it known to the patients and their families that the hospice exists and tell them what the hospice can do for them.

   I think the marvelous thing about hospice is the attention and concern. Sometimes when a patient is diagnosed as terminal, the attention goes to someone who is not terminal. And the terminal patient is kind of left alone. He doesn't get the same attention.

E M   You mean attention from the medical staff? The nursing staff?

R H   Yes. And for a patient who is terminal to have somebody to care for him and treat him in a dignified manner and make life comfortable is wonderful. I don't see why the hospice shouldn't survive.

E M   Did anything about the hospice surprise you?

R H   When I went into the hospice program, I discovered that there were so many young people in it. Young people often don't seem to think about dying or about helping people who are dying. But there are quite a number of young people in the program. I think one fellow is only twenty-four. I know that there is one girl who is very young. I think she's a school teacher. She is very interested in the program because she has had to take care of her mother and father and she has been inspired to help other people in these conditions. So it isn't just a gray lady type of thing. The volunteers are working people. Yet they make time to devote — their spare time — which is a remarkable thing.

Chapter 11

"HOSPICE WORK CAME NATURALLY"

DIALOGUE WITH TWO VOLUNTEERS

Vivian and Richard Handel are hospice volunteers. He's a salesman; she's an eighth-grade school teacher. Over the years, both singly and together, they have cared for terminally ill family members and friends. They have seen the shortcomings and felt the frustration of the traditional care given to patients who are dying. The Handels talk here about their hospice work and about many of the experiences that led to it.

R H   We have been assigned a patient. The two of us are working on a case together, which involves a gentleman named Rudy, who has ALS [amyotrophic lateral sclerosis], commonly called Lou Gehrig's disease. It's a neurological disease. And he's had it about a year-and-a-half. He was a crane operator. Worked in the steel mills.

This gentleman can't communicate in any way other than with his eyes or with some sounds. You can't understand him when he attempts to speak. He has no movement of his limbs. But he can hear and he can see and he can think. He understands absolutely everything.

V H   We have to be very careful, we have found, not to talk around Rudy. We talk to him. We include him in the conversation.

R H   Rudy is cared for by his wife, Chris, and his two children, ages six and seven.

V H   He is 46 or 47. His wife is much younger. She's 27, she told me.

R H   Somehow or other, the communication between Rudy and

his wife and the two kids is almost telepathic.

V H The children are so attuned to his needs and to his wants that they function just beautifully with him. I don't know what's going to happen later, but right now, it's an amazing thing.

R H We know, medically speaking, he is terminal. But he could live for God knows how long. ALS is not like cancer. He may not die of ALS. He probably will die of respiratory problems. He might choke to death. Or he might drown in his own saliva. Or he might get pneumonia.

V H Before we got involved with the patient, we were very privileged to have the neurologist in charge of the ALS clinic at Billings invite us to come down there. We spent one whole afternoon with the staff. They all talked with us and gave us a world of information. We were also given reading material on ALS patients and their care.

That was so important, because the patient's wife is no longer able to bring him into the clinic. It's too much of a problem now because he can't function in any way on his own. She must move him bodily in every way. And also, the hospital doesn't have a ramp near the ALS clinic to make it possible for her to get the wheelchair into the clinic.

It's just been a terrible effort for her. That was why they suggested that he would benefit from hospice care. His wife could come and get anything she needed for him, but even that was becoming increasingly difficult. So that's how we got into this case.

The doctor has explained to us that if Rudy has to be hospitalized, his wife would have to stay with him in order to communicate with him because nobody else would know what he wanted. His family is so tuned in to him that they just pick it all up.

R H The other day when we were there, Rudy's brother came over. And Rudy let his daughter know that there was someting he wanted to say. So she started with the alphabet. She called off the alphabet because he is able to let her know the letters in the words so that she can form the words and phrases.

V H   Now this child is in second grade.

R H   It turned out that Rudy wanted to make sure that his
       brother was offered a beer. So she turned to her uncle and
       said, "Daddy wants to know if you want a beer." He said,
       "Yeah, sure." So she went to the refrigerator and got him
       a beer.

V H   In the beginning, we asked ourselves just what it was that
       we could do for them. What would be of help in this situa-
       tion. And we found that the help is not only for the patient
       in this situation, it is also for the family. They are the ones
       who have more of the unmet needs.

E M   What kinds of things do you do for Rudy and Chris and the
       kids?

V H   We've done such a variety of things. We found, for example,
       that Rudy is a baseball fan — a Cub fan. And he was very
       interested in a specific player who was new to the Cubs. So
       Dick called the Cubs and told them about Rudy. And they
       said, "Oh, we can send him a get well card, if you would
       like." But we said, "You'd better hold off for a while."
       Then we called the doctor to ask whether it was all right for
       them to send a get well card, because he isn't ever going
       to get well. But the doctor said, "Oh, absolutely. It's per-
       fectly in order. He may be better today than he was on sev-
       eral other days — so that's better!" It was just a simple
       thing, sending a card.

E M   Has it been sent?

R H   Oh, yes.

V H   Oh, yes. He has it proudly displayed there.

R H   The kids make sure that everyone who comes in gets to see
       the card that the Chicago Cubs sent to their father. If they
       don't show it to them, Rudy will remind them to show it.
       He's very proud of the fact that he got a card from the
       Cubs.

V H   We have also been able to facilitate getting some equipment
       he has needed. He has been very fortunate. He had been
       referred to Billings by his local hospital, which did not have
       the facilities to care for him. As a result, through the ser-
       vices of the ALS clinic at Billings, he has been receiving

many different kinds of aids from Muscular Dystrophy, Easter Seals, and a variety of other agencies.

We've also helped to facilitate getting new equipment, because he's needed new equipment. He needed a neck brace, because it's too tiring for him to try to hold up his head. He can't control it. His wife wanted to get a head pointer to use with an alphabet board, and a harness so that she could take him out in the wheelchair. He likes to go out. He has a reclining wheelchair but she feels more secure when he's in a harness so he won't slide out. Then he needed some lamb's wool padding for the bed. A lap board has also been ordered for him.

As his condition deteriorates — and it's deteriorating rapidly — he needs different things. His wife has a blender and fixes all of his food in the blender. He is still able to eat what she fixes that way. But tube feeding comes next. And she may or may not be able to do it.

They had told us how he would be fed, but I've never been there when it happened. You've been there, though, Dick.

R H   Yes, I've been there a couple of times when he's been fed. It's not an appetizing thing to see. Ninety percent of the food gets on his bib. Only 10 percent gets down. It's a situation in which you finish the food on the plate and then you start with the food on the bib.

V H   At one point, Chris told me that one of her problems was keeping Rudy in good spirits. So we asked her if he liked to read. She said yes, he did like to read. Now Rudy has a Spanish surname, so we assumed that they were Spanish. And we called and got all kinds of information about books and magazines in Spanish for the physically handicapped. Then we found out that Chris doesn't even understand Spanish, that her mother was Polish. But Rudy is Mexican. It's interesting how you assume things that don't necessarily happen to be so.

Anyway, we found that there are things available through the library for incapacitated people. As long as he was not able to turn pages of a book, he was eligible for things that are provided on tapes or records. It's amazing what the library provides for you. Dick went down and picked it all up and brought it out to them.

R H   They provide a cassette player or they provide a record player and they provide all of the periodicals, all of the books on tapes or records. They have a catalogue of cassettes that must be two and one-half inches thick. The library also supplies you with an advisor. They give you a telephone number and a name. Then you call that person and tell them that you would like to have such and such books — either on records or on tapes — and they put it in the mail to you so it's delivered to your home. When you're finished, all you do is turn the label over on the container, put the tape or record in the container, and drop it in the mailbox with no postage due. You are supplied continually with whatever you want.

V H   With as much as you want. We found that Rudy is interested in science fiction, mysteries, and things like that. So these were the kinds of things we got for him.

E M   Do you just use your initiative in finding these resources and services?

V H   Yes, but much of it we learned from his wife, much of it we learned from the clinic, and much of it we were told by friends.

E M   The library service, for example.

V H   I knew about that. I just wasn't sure that he would qualify. Now I find out that they are going to make this service available to all ALS patients because they would all qualify.

E M   Because of your efforts in his behalf?

V H   Yes. You have to have a physician's statement. You have to have the medical basis to receive all of these things. Dick went down to the hospital and got the statement.

These tapes are just another way for him to pass the time, to provide change, and to relieve Chris for a limited amount of time.

Another thing that the patient's wife wanted was a telephone answering machine. And we couldn't understand why. But it's because she takes the children to school — just a couple of blocks away — and she's afraid someone will call and she will miss some important information.

R H Also, Rudy gets very upset when he hears the phone because he can't answer it. The longer the phone rings, the more upset he becomes and the more agitated he becomes. And there's no way for him to release his agitation. He gets very frustrated.

V H Anyhow, Dick got her a phone answering machine. And this is the light of her life. She feels she's not missing anything and the phone doesn't ring long enough to disturb him.

Another thing that the doctor suggested was a speaker phone, an amplifier. But we found them to be very, very expensive. And I don't think it will be possible for them. Dick contacted the telephone company. There are a lot of phones for handicapped persons. But he can't use any of them. There are pillow-activated phones and breath-activated phones and all kinds of phones. But he can't use any of them. Somebody has to be there to answer the phone. But he could listen to the conversation with an amplifying phone. We'll just have to see if we can find some funding for an amplifier.

E M How long have you been involved with Rudy and his wife and his children?

V H About two months, two and one-half months. We've become sort of a liaison with the clinic for the two of them. The doctor calls us. He checks with us periodically and we often relay messages. In fact, the last clinic appointment she had, we had set up in a roundabout way. Dick went down to the hospital and talked to the staff. He told them what the situation was and that he thought it was time for her to come in so they could get some information from her.

We didn't know what her plans were in case he started to choke and she couldn't do anything about it. We had talked to her once about this.

R H Vivian and I had been talking to Chris about what she would do when an emergency should arise. Did she know that she could call us and she should call the doctor and the hospital. She should *not* call 911. If she called 911, the ambulance would take him to the nearest hospital. And the nearest hospital would not be able to care for him properly.

And Chris said, "That's true. I know I don't call 911. And if Rudy ever gets sick, I'll have to call a private ambulance and take him to Billings. If he should ever get sick, that's what I would do." I'm looking at my wife and she's picking up on it too. We didn't say anything until we got to the car. Then I said to Vivian, "What the hell's the matter with her? The guy is dead on his feet, and she's saying, 'Yes, if he gets sick . . .' "

V H   You see, she doesn't consider him sick. Literally, the man is completely incapacitated, and she doesn't look at him as sick.

R H   He's not sick. As long as he can eat, as long as he can sit up, as long as he can watch television, as long as he can communicate with her — he's not sick.

E M   Is that because she is so young?

V H   No, we understand this is characteristic of families of ALS patients.

E M   Do the two of you always go together to see him?

V H   No.

E M   Does she call you when she needs things or do you check in with her on a regular basis?

R H   We check in with her and she has called us on a couple of occasions. As often as is helpful to them, but it's a situation in which you cannot impose yourself upon them. Until she is ready to accept more help from us, we just have to wait.

V H   Friday was the first time that she would leave us alone with him, because she had a clinic appointment. I think she has had some bad experiences with other people who were helping. She said she has had some home health aides who would come in. And when she had to go away, she would come back and find him alone. They didn't wait for her. So she's been very reluctant. But Friday, we finally passed the test, I guess.

R H   We talk to her perhaps three times a week. We call her up on the phone and say, "Hi, Chris, how are you doing? What do you need? Is there anything we can do for you?"

V H We usually try to tie the conversation into something we have talked about before.

R H And we've made a point of being there at least once a week, if for no other reason than just to stop in and say, "Hello." We always call before we go and say, "I'm going to be in the neighborhood Friday, and if it's alright with you, I'll stop by." She'll always say, "Yes, yes, come on over."

The children look on us now as friends. And they're excited when we come to visit. They take it as friends coming to visit. But we watch ourselves so as not to presume on the relationship. We asked Chris whether it would be all right to buy something for the children for Easter. She thought that would be fine. So I had some of my kids at school make Easter baskets that we filled with candy and brought over. We found out — after Easter — that they were the only things they had received.

V H These children are so involved in their father's care that we really question how they're going to function later.

R H This is something that we're going to have to bring up at the patient care conference with Jean, who is head of the Bereavement Committee of our hospice. When Rudy does pass away, it's going to be a fantastic load off of Chris, physically, but it's going to create such a void in her life and in the lives of these two children that somehow or other something is going to have to be done to help them over it.

V H I think it's going to be difficult. The fact is that the children are so involved in his care that when he does die, they will be without the center of their lives.

E M Do the children have friends of their own? Do they play at all?

R H They have friends at school.

V H They play at school and outside sometimes. Now the Friday we were there, they came and told us that their mother had said they couldn't go out to play until she came home. They said they sure hoped that she would come home early enough so they could go outside. It happened to be a nice day.

E M It's being quite an experience, isn't it?

V H Amazingly so. To be very honest with you, when we first thought of becoming involved with the hospice, I said to Dick, "I have to wait and see how this is going to affect us. Is it going to be something in which we can really be of some help or are we going to be so devastated that we're not going to be able to do anything but cry with them." I don't think that's so terrible, because they know that you care. But we didn't want to not be able to be of help.

E M How do you feel about it now?

R H It's no problem at all. There was not a problem for me to begin with. And I wouldn't call it a problem for Vivian, it was just a well-taken thought. I said, "Look, go through the training. You haven't signed your life away. You can stop any time, if you want to." When it came time for her to say, "Okay, it's all right," she had been through the training and had come to terms with herself. So she could say "Yes, it's all right for me."

　　I think our volunteer coordinator was very hesitant about giving Rudy's case to us because of the devastation that might have been involved.

V H She didn't want to stop us right at the beginning.

R H Right. I think we might have surprised her a little bit because it has not had that kind of an effect on either one of us.

V H You sure count your blessings, every time you come home from there.

R H Yes, because we have seen as bad as our coordinator might have thought it would be.

V H You never know the point at which it is going to be more than you can take. But it hasn't come for me yet.

E M Do you think that this particular illness is as bad as you will see? Can you think of anything worse than this kind of illness?

V H I can't. I really can't. There may be something, but I can't think what it could be right now.

E M So if you can deal with this, you can deal with almost any case you might have.

R H   Cancer's not nice to look at. It's not easy to be with. And I understand that the majority of cases that are referred to the hospice are cancer cases. In our training program, they just fleetingly mentioned neurological diseases. And boom, here we are.

V H   If it works out the way we think — all of our volunteers are out now — I may pair up with someone else on a new case. Rudy's on a plateau and Dick's able to meet the needs.

E M   What's the new case?

V H   It's a cancer patient. She's a seventy-six-year-old woman and her husband is approximately the same age. She has a terminal cancer now. She has had it for a number of years, but it has metastasized now and she is not really able to function anymore. She is very angry at her husband for not "carrying the load," as she puts it. Now it's hard to say whether he does or he doesn't. You have to sift things out.

    Evidently, she really feels that she has still been taking care of the house and he doesn't do a damn thing, that he hasn't done a thing for thirty-five or forty years. She has a lot of hostility and, evidently, she's in a lot of pain.

    If I took this case, I would have to depend on the other volunteer a lot — there are two to a case — because if it turns out that Rudy and Chris are needing more things, I feel that I would want to go back to them. I don't want Rudy and his family to feel that I am walking out on them.

E M   Why did you become involved in hospice work?

V H   Over the years we have both been very committed to caring for a variety of people that we have been very close to. So hospice is something that came to us quite naturally.

E M   Before you got involved, had you known of someone who had had hospice care?

V H   No. But we knew some that should have had it. We realized, in so many ways, the voids that were in the present system. For example, Dick went to see a friend of ours — a little over a year ago, wasn't it? This young man had cancer of the pancreas. It's very fast moving and he had to be hospitalized at the end.

    The man was divorced and had a college age child, who

was away, and an aged mother. He stayed with his niece and her family. All of those things kept closing in on him. The family didn't know where to turn for help. The only things they knew were that they could not leave him alone and that they wanted him to be with those who cared for him. It was touch and go for everybody. Not just for the patient, but for the family. It was a most traumatic experience.

At the end he was hospitalized. So Dick went to see him in the hospital. The man was in terrible pain. We couldn't understand why he would have to be in such pain. We thought there should have been something that the hospital could do for him. But they go according to the book.

It didn't change until Dick got hold of a resident physician who was able to change things. He said, "There's no reason why he should be like that. They can put the pain medication in the IV and he can be constantly pain free." Doing that made all of the difference for him, for this family, for everybody. But how many people have the opportunity to do something about a situation like that? And our friend was in a first-class hospital. But they have their rules.

E M   You said that over the years you have cared for people who were very close to you.

V H   Yes, I was married previously. My first husband died of cancer. We had a very young family, but we had people around us who provided all of the supportive care. I know that I would not have been able to function without it. If such a thing happened today, we would not have that many to call on, even though we have many very dear friends. Our family has diminished. There are different stages in your life and you have different people available to help you.

E M   Were you caring for these poeple in their homes?

R H   Yes. In most instances. At least the majority of the time. Vivian's sister, who lived one house away, passed away at home. She had a nurse, but Vivian and her husband and various members of the family and friends were actually functioning as "hospice volunteers," without knowing that was what it was. After Janet passed away, other members of the family became ill and passed away. And friends of ours, too. We just carried it through, doing it naturally.

As Vivian says, we have been "hospice people" without being connected with a hospice for many, many years.

Chapter 12

"IN THE HANDS, HEARTS, AND HOMES
OF THOSE WHO CARE"

DIALOGUE WITH FOUR HOSPICE CAREGIVERS

The oncology unit in Little Company of Mary Hospital, Evergreen Park, Illinois, is the base of operation for the hospital's hospice program. One quiet afternoon, members of its committed team — Shirley Oberg, R.N., director, Oncology Nursing Practice; Louis Mallon, R.N., Hospice Nurse Coordinator; Sister Roseann McCarthy, hospice pastoral care representative; and Judy Lickteig, A.C.S.W. — shared their thoughts, feelings, and questions about their work and their involvements.

R H   How did Little Company of Mary happen to start a hospice program?

S R M   We're a nursing community. We were founded in England and our Mother House is in Rome. Our primary mission is prayer for and care of the sick and dying. We started in home nursing and gradually progressed, seeing needs change, from home nursing to institutional nursing. And now we're seeing it change again, this time to a kind of combination of home nursing and hospital nursing.

L M   As far as the hospice itself is concerned, it is my understanding that one of our administrators, who visited Rome and talked to the Mother General, was told to come back and start a hospice in the United States.

R H   What's the focus of your program?

S O   The focus is in the community. It's a home care program. Sometime in the future — as part of our long-range plan — we hope to start an in-hospital hospice. We do not now

140

have any hospice beds in the hospital. Right now, if our patients need to be admitted, they are admitted to an acute-care bed in the hospital.

R H   So you care for all of your patients at home.

L M   Yes, and I think it has worked out well. We have had about sixty patients in the program over the last two years. And we've had only about twelve that we have had to return to the hospital — either for pain control or symptom control or when families could not cope with having the patient die at home.

R H   You deal daily with pain, fear, and anxiety, don't you?

S O   Yes. But I think the very fact that hospice care is patient-family centered relieves a lot of anxiety in the patients and in their families. They know that they will deal with the hospice team, that they won't have to call an answering service and not know when the doctor is going to respond. I think that has reduced a lot of the anxiety.

S R M   When the family is supported through the team, it can cope with most things better. Then family members are able to keep the patient at home, where the patient wants to be. They have the hotline, they have the team to call on, and they have other resources that give them security.

R H   Do you find that you get support back from patients and families?

L M   Oh, yes. I think patients are prepared far in advance. They are ready to die and they are waiting for the family to be ready. Because of this, patients are a support not only to their families but also to the team.

J L   There's no question that we get a lot of support and strength from helping families at a crucial time. But we're not doing all the giving; we receive a lot from families in return. The support we receive from one another helps. We can use one another's strength as back-up.

R H   What personal satisfaction do you get out of your work?

J L   I have a sense of satisfaction in working with patients and families in a crisis time in their lives. Just recently, a woman came to me who was very upset because she knew that her husband was dying and she had hoped to share her feelings with him. For some reason, he did not want to share with her. Somehow, I was able to facilitate open discussion between the two of them, allowing them time to share what was on their minds. And that was a good feeling.

Personally, that is the greatest satisfaction — coming into a situation where there's a crisis in the family, when people are already mourning and grieving. They started doing that when the diagnosis was given. We're intervening in a situation in which the people are predisposed to intervention and are saying, "Yes, we accept your help." There are those, of course, who chose not to.

R H   What do you do when someone is a little reluctant to accept your help?

J L   I think we have to allow them a little bit of time and space. When families are hesitant to say, "We're ready to accept your help," my position is to give them time to think it over. There are so many things going on in their lives. They are trying to come to grips with the fact that someone is going to die.

Some people choose to do their own grieving and provide their own private support. And they don't need us. I think we have to acknowledge this. We have to allow them to choose, to say "No." People don't have to accept our intervention because we offer it.

R H   Shirley, would you like to share some of your experiences?

S O   There's such a difference between the terminal patient in a hospital and a terminal patient in his home. In the hospital, we more or less outline what patient and family can do during this terminal stage. In the hospice program, they tell us what they want to do. We work with the family and we do whatever we can to be supportive of them. We work with the family to see that we are meeting the needs of both the patient and the family — not meeting the needs of the building or the institution. I think you see that in the way that families are able to cope at a time like this.

R H   What happens when things go sour?

S O   Go sour in the home?

R H   In the home.

S O   I don't think things go sour in the home. Sometimes situations occur that are totally overwhelming. But I can't say that's going sour, because I have always had the help of the other members of the hospice team available.

Not long ago, I found myself in a situation like that. And it was because Sister Roseann and Judy joined me that I was able to continue in my role of being supportive to the family. I can't think of anything ever going sour because I always have the team available to assist me.

J L   There have been times in the past that I have questioned — after a patient had died — whether or not hospice intervention had been beneficial to that family. I'm thinking of a situation in which the patient was home for just a short period of time. Things seemed rather rushed and chaotic in the home, and the family didn't quite understand who we were and what we were all about. There are times like that when I question whether or not it was appropriate to get involved.

S O   Maybe it's a question of getting involved sooner. If it's just a matter of two weeks, what benefit is hospice?

J L   Would they have been better off without us?

S R M In a situation like this, you are really asking the family to adjust to new people coming into their lives. They are having to extend themselves and cope with you and relate to you on a social level when they are really not up to it.

There's one situation that I can think of in which I came into the picture really at the terminal moment. I felt like the family was trying to extend itself to me and I wanted to extend myself to them.

R H   Was it only in the final stage that you became involved with the patient?

S R M Yes, it was about the last visit. The family's needs were being met by their parish group. I came in because the parish priest was on vacation and was going to be away.

It was for a specific purpose that I was there. I was able to carry that out. But normally I would have had the opportunity to be more involved and supportive.

R H   You seem to have a little apprehension about that situation. Did you fear getting involved?

S R M   No, I would like to have been involved. It's just that these people had to go out of their way to welcome me or greet me and be sociable. If I had been part of the process, I wouldn't have been a stranger coming in at the last minute. They just seemed to be pulling energies out of themselves to extend themselves to me. Normally, there's a slow process of building a relationship.

When Judy was talking earlier, it struck me how we really do try to respect where the individuals are and respect their need for privacy. We have had people say, "I only want the nurse with me," or "I could use the social service person," or "You might ask the sister in pastoral care to stop by." They're free to choose the person they relate to.

We've seen that recently in families we've been involved with. One person in one family chose Judy, one person chose me, one chose Louise, one chose Shirley, and one chose the volunteer. There was a complement of ministry there. We're working *with* each other. We're not vying with each other, not trying to see who can give them the most help.

S O   There are no territorial rights. I think there are gray areas in our work. Yet when we know that we might be getting into a gray area — in pastoral services or social service, for example — we will very easily say something about it to the family and then the most involved person will come in.

R H   What is the most important thing you have gotten out of your work?

S R M   I think it is being aware of people's needs, being able to bring something to offer, in the sense of support, and being there with them. After offering the support and sensing mutualness in the relationship, I feel sometimes a completeness or a wholeness in myself.

To me, this work is also an extension of the church. It's the fact that someone cares. It's not imposing my beliefs, but accepting people where they're at. It's a sense of being in a relationship that is profound. It's the recognition of being on sacred ground with another person. And I sense that person's vulnerability and I sense my own vulnerability, too. I really feel touched by the people I'm caring for and they feel touched by me. That's very fulfilling, but it can be very draining.

To other people it is a human involvement, not a religious involvement. But, again, it's caring for another person.

L M   I think the greatest satisfaction is in knowing that you're helping the patient and family to cope with the situation. And I think one of the other things is the privilege you are allowed by the patient and the family to share in the illness and in their pain and in their feelings — their inner feelings about what is going on. It's in giving the family the support it needs and in caring for the patient, giving the patient the support he needs.

Most of the time we find that the patient is ready to die far sooner than the family is ready to accept it. And we help the patient's family work through that. With the support they receive, they are able to accept the situation. As Judy mentioned before, they are talking to us and letting us know that they are already grieving. The patient grieves for himself and his loss and the family is grieving for the patient. There's a different atmosphere when a patient dies at home than there is when he dies in the hospital. There's a quiet and calm acceptance.

R H   What's the biggest drain on you as a hospice worker?

S O   I think that it is when I have been with the patient when he died. And I am grieving. My family is supportive to me, but I think this is the group — the hospice team — that is most supportive. When I grieve, they allow me the opportunity to verbalize my grief. And I find that is very human and very helpful.

J L   After having worked with a patient and gotten very close to him, I find the need to do my own grieving. I'm part of the bereavement team that follows the family through bereavement and the conflict I have is wanting to keep in touch with all of them. Yet that's not possible. The hardest part for me is to terminate one relationship and then be as invested, energetic, and enthusiastic in picking up a new patient and family as I have been working with the others.

L M   I would agree with Shirley and Judy. One of the most draining and hardest times is when a patient dies. Of course, it all depends on how long you've had the patient in the program and how close you've become with the patient and the family. There are days you come in here and you're just completely washed out. You can't do anything. You can't even sit down and think. It takes a couple of days — sometimes a couple of weeks — before you actually feel the same way you did before — all inspired to keep going on.

And sometimes it depends on how many deaths you have had in a short period of time. That takes a great toll at times. Sometimes we've had two or three deaths in a matter of only a couple of days. And each one drains you out completely. But you always have the support of the team.

I know I've found that, sometimes, at home I have been positively drained. And at the time I felt I was getting support from my family. But I wasn't getting as much as I really wanted, because my family was not grieving like I was. My family had known about the patient, but they were not experiencing that same type of grief. It's not until you get back to the team that you get the support you need. Everyone is in the same situation, grieving with you.

J L   We get our support from one another because we're all involved, but how long can we continue doing that? At some point, we'll need to go outside our group for support, and bring back renewed strength. You can't keep drawing on people who are continuously giving. You can't keep doing that forever.

S R M I agree with what has been said. But what I find even more difficult is realizing that, when someone has died, there's a person left behind with a whole lot of pain. Now, I make only one, maybe two, follow-up visits. I encourage that person to see the bereavement social worker rather than to see me.

I find having to let go of that person very difficult. People still call me and often the social worker says, "So and so wants to talk to you, could you give them a call." I do that, but I continue by phone instead of going to see them. Burnout is a real thing.

R H You all seem to be telling me that you're having trouble with empathy versus sympathy.

S O We did have that problem recently. The patient was a staff member we all knew. And that may have made us sympathetic. But I will have to say that, in this case, I think we did have a tendency to bend toward sympathy. But we tried to be empathetic in order to give this family strength. I don't think you could have helped but identify with someone you have worked with, someone who is your own age.

She died the day before Memorial Day. And I think that some of the feelings you are hearing from us today are caused by the fact that this is so fresh in our minds. She was one of us. She worked on this unit. It had a big impact on all of us.

S R M There is another patient that we were especially close to. I think the family situation with John was so unusual. We saw such commitment on the family's part, it seemed to infuse all of us with commitment.

J L How do you keep from becoming involved? I've gotten "over-involved" in the past and then found myself having to pull back for a while. I guess we all have our own survival techniques.

S R M What makes a difference to me is that the *hospice team* really *does care* about the patient and family. We encourage one another and challenge each other to grow in wholeness.

Hospice is an alive program! Hospice is in the hands, the hearts, and the homes of those who care. It is a tremendous support to patients and families. I *believe* in hospice.

Chapter 13

"THE TERRIBLE LONELINESS OF IT"

DIALOGUE WITH A VOLUNTEER

After neurosurgery, when she lay isolated and alone, Jean Knoll thought she was dying. And she was struck by the horror of dying alone, of having no one notice and no one care. Through the miracle of modern medicine, she not only survived, she recovered. But the painful memory of her near brush with death — and the circumstances surrounding it — are with her still. Because of this, she brings to her work as a hospice volunteer some very special insights. Jean Knoll talks about her illness, the changes it made in her life, her thoughts on quality of life, and what she can bring to her hospice patients.

J K   For a long time, the headaches I was getting had been written off as tension headaches. My protestations to the contrary, the headaches continued to be dismissed as just psychosomatic.

    I can remember, particularly, when my neck began to swell — before it actually ruptured. I went to the doctor I was then seeing, put his hand on the back of my neck, and said, "Feel that. That is not psychosomatic. There's something wrong with my neck." He told me that my neck muscles were the tightest, tensest muscles he had ever felt. I threw a paperweight at him and left. At that point, when I had physical evidence that something was indeed wrong and when I couldn't get anyone to hear that, I began to perceive that I might, in fact, be dying. And because my condition didn't fit into somebody's category, I might not ever really be heard about my pain.

    Shortly after that incident, my neck did rupture. I woke

149

up one morning and couldn't move on one side and I had a lot of trouble moving my tongue. The first thing I thought was that I had had a stroke. It was ultimately diagnosed that the disc that had been breaking apart all those years had finally given way and the second and third vertebrae had collapsed onto each other. Fortunately for me, it involved the left side of my body and my tongue, not the crucial parts of me. Then, sure enough, everybody took me seriously. I was sick. The doctors weren't sure, however, how much could be done to undo the damage. They made no promises that they were going to be able to do too much more than stabilize my neck after that.

I remember being very angry that I had been in pain for so long without anybody to listen to it and to treat it with any kind of dignity. Pain, if it is not yours, is easy to dismiss. At the time, I was taking a lot of pain medication. And I remember a lot of sermons coming out of the mouths of doctors to the effect that taking all this medication was not good. But the quality of my life was so poor that, without it, I spent every day in bed. I remember making the decision for myself that whatever the long-range effects of the medicine were, the short-term effects would make whatever time I had left at least bearable.

R H   Did you feel at the time that you were going to die?

J K   I wasn't sure, but I thought it was a distinct possibility.

R H   You acted under the assumption that this might be a fatal illness.

J K   My father had a history of brain aneurysms and I had every reason to believe that that was exactly what was going on in my own head.

R H   How old were you at the time?

J K   Twenty-five. The other memory, aside from the memory of all that rage, was the memory of the terrible loneliness of it. I watched people who cared for me, who saw me get sicker, and who could get no more response from the doctors than I did, pull back because they didn't know what to do. And I remember the most horrible part of the experience being that I might die and nobody would notice or care. And when I lay in traction in the intensive care ward after they operated on my neck, I can remember thinking that I could just die in that bed and for everybody concerned it would be a big relief. They wouldn't have to face it anymore.

The notion is still so horrible to me, of dying alone without anybody to say, "I know it hurts and I'm sorry. It's terrible and it's not fair. And I'll not preach to you any more, I'll just hold your hand."

I made a very strong decision to go to a hospice if I were clearly not going to go any further. I realized that the decision about the quality of my life, for here and now and for whatever time was left, was mine to make. Miraculously I began to get well. It took me a good year to realize that it wasn't a temporary improvement. But I was still desperately sick. I weighed ninety-eight pounds by the end of the year.

R H You're a hospice volunteer, aren't you?

J K Yes.

R H Do you bring some of the experiences you had to caring for patients?

J K All of them, I think. I bring my sense that death is not the worst thing that can happen, but that for everyone involved, the process of dying can be an agonizing one and that meeting death with any kind of equanimity is not foolish or insane. It is a fact of release for the patient and for those that the patient loves. It's a peculiarly hopeless, yet a kind of hopeful, process.

I guess I bring to them my sense of the immediacy related to the quality of life I have now. Tomorrow morning, I may wake and that side of my body may not work again. That says to me that what time is left should be filled with kindness, caring, and honesty. It also says to me that suffering is much more profitably shared.

R H You said you made a strong decision that you would go to a hospice if you weren't going to go any further. Why did you make that decision?

J K Because it would be an enormous relief to have somebody here to talk to about dying — someone who wouldn't cringe. An enormous relief to have someone saying, "I know what you mean, the quality of your life, today and tomorrow, is what matters when the quantity of your life is uncertain." An enormous relief to have with me people who spend some time thinking about dying, who are not so horrified by the whole concept, so that when I come to terms with death for my own self, I can express what I learn and what I feel and what I don't understand — and not have people flinch.

R H   You're saying that often members of the medical team are frightened by the subject of death, that they run from it?

J K   Yes. They can't look at it. And the patient who says, "I think I'm dying," and family members who say, "I think my loved one is dying," are just dismissed.

R H   What do you think causes that?

J K   I don't know. I think it's partly just the experience of medical training — the experience that encourages people to concentrate too much on making the patient well. I think if you don't cooperate and, in fact, don't get well, you are, somehow, a bad patient. And you are somewhat less interesting than you would be if you, in fact, responded in interesting ways to interesting therapies. I think part of it is also that people who are medical professionals, in most cases, lead an emotionally isolated life. Many of them have never seen death. We live in a society where the dying are put away, the way the insane used to be.

R H   That is really vivid in your mind — the feeling that you were put away when you thought you might be dying.

J K   Yes, absolutely. I thought that I was going to die and that nobody would notice. I was a name and I connected a bunch of tests together — tests that didn't prove very much of anything to anybody, even though I kept saying, "I hurt."

R H   What do you feel you can bring to the dying patient?

J K   The sense that the most horrible part of death is not the act of dying, but the loneliness of it. If we ever need the comfort of our fellow human beings and of those we love and care about, it is at the point that we're pulling together the last days and weeks of our lives.

R H Are you still angry about your experience?

J K You bet I am. I'm in the process of seeing my mother die right now. So this is all very close. Three months ago, when I told the doctors I was taking my mother home to die, they laughed. Four days later I brought her back to the emergency room in a coma. Then one young doctor came out of the room and said her blood sugar was low. He said that to me in the hall. I took him by the shoulders, turned him round, and pushed him back into the room. I said, "Look at her. This is not a woman with low blood sugar. This is a woman in a coma. She's been like this for days. Look at her." Not only does he deny the evidence of his own senses, but also the evidence of someone else's. I don't think I want to get rid of my personal pain about this kind of experience.

R H You want to help other people make the transition without having the pain you had to experience.

J K Without the loneliness, without the anger. Maybe without some of the sense of desperation. I'm sure that one doesn't ever die without feeling desperate at some point in the process, especially if the process goes on for a long time. Dying persons need someone who will listen to them when they say they feel desperate.

R H Were you alienated from your family too?

J K Yes. They got no support from the medical community in believing that I was sick. I think that a lot of what they looked at and saw in me was psychosomatic — until the day my left arm and leg didn't work. It was much easier for them to look at it that way than to look at undiagnosed pain and try to make sense out of it. It hurts to see someone you care about hurt. And when you can dismiss it, somehow, and have the doctors' blessing in the process, why not?

R H It must be very frustrating to be experiencing what you were experiencing without any kind of support or understanding or human intervention.

J K It's not fair to say *without any*, but without a whole lot of it, without nearly enough to have made very much difference.

After I had had the surgery, I was in a neck brace and weighed ninety-eight pounds. The doctor who did the surgery encouraged me to take walks to get my strength back. And he suggested that I go to the Baskin-Robbins ice cream shop every day, if I could get there, eat until I was full, and turn around and come home. The first day I got all the way to Baskin-Robbins, the neurosurgeon who had put his hand on my neck and told me those were terribly tense muscles four days before my neck ruptured was there with his kids. Earlier, I had asked my neurosurgeon to write to him and explain to him what they had done when they went in there. And I believed he had. The doctor in Baskin-Robbins looked at me in this little getup of foam rubber and metal and all. Then he said, "Well, did that operation help or are you still getting those terrible tension headaches?" I dropped my ice cream on his shin, because I couldn't think of what to say. He ignored even the evidence after the fact that I had had chipped bones in my neck. There was hard cold evidence that he wouldn't look at because it didn't fit the pattern.

R H   The absurdity of the responses really blows your mind, doesn't it?

J K   It's incredible. My mother is, was then, and will be for a while yet, dying. And yet the physician made that remark about the blood sugar. They can't see it. They don't understand it. What can't be understood, what can't be comprehended rationally, must not be real.

R H   What was the most humiliating thing that happened to you during your illness?

J K   To be told that it was my fault. To be told that taking medicine to kill the pain — pain that I had made up in the first place out of my own poor adjustment to life — was evidence of further weakness in my character and personality. To be told that it was my responsibility to clean up my act to fit somebody else's picture of how I ought to be. To have doctors *tell me what I felt* instead of *asking me how I felt* and listening to me. I think those things were the worst.

R H   How do you feel about the professionals who are involved in hospice care?

J K   I don't interact enough with them as professionals to make a very informed judgement about the quality of care and concern that they offer. But what I am always impressed by is the sense that there is just a pathetic handful of professional people who understand that it hurts and who care that it hurts.

R H   You've used that word "care" a number of times. Obviously it is significant to you.

J K   It represents the difference between saying, "Yes, I understand in my head that this is a painful process, I recognize a painful process as I sit here and see that you weigh ninety-eight pounds and see your family in grief beside you" — the difference between that and saying, "God, that's awful, I'm sorry. What can I do to help a little bit? I can't fix it, but maybe I can make it a little easier."

R H   How do you see your role as a hospice volunteer?

J K   As a good neighbor and as a sensitive friend. Somebody who's been on both sides of that bed and, maybe, has a little bit to share as a result.

R H   What do you think will happen to the hospice movement?

J K   My great hope, of course, is that it will become an option that everyone knows about and understands, and an option that will not be as costly as it is for so many people. Both of these are obvious hopes. I suppose I have a greater hope that, as the hospice gains respectability, gains in stature in the medical and nonmedical community, its insights into the humanity of people who suffer and die can be applied to all care given — particularly to the care of the aged.

The aged are often not "terminal," but someone who is eighty-five years old doesn't necessarily have a whole lot of time left. So the quality of the time that is left to the aged, however infirm, is something that needs some long, hard looking at and thinking about. I guess the notion of warehousing someone at any point in a human life, without facing the implications of that warehousing for the human being and for his or her family, is a blind and half-assed way to treat people, who are too old or too sick to scream about it.

R H   What would you change about the hospice concept?

J K   I find it very problematic that one must have the *diagnosis* of terminal illness before one can be admitted to a hospice. It seems to me that the real question is one of the consciousness of dying. My mother has a consciousness of dying. I have a consciousness of her dying. I think a hospice would be an enormously helpful thing for her — to have people tend to her pain and listen to her cry — but because she has an undiagnosed and untreatable disease, she is *not diagnosed* as terminal. Because it can't be documented — although she clearly is terminal — she can't be admitted to a hospice. I hope that will be changed sometime in the future. When I was sick, I wouldn't have been admitted to a hospice either. I couldn't have gotten a doctor to sign the piece of paper.

I would like to see hospices give weight to the patient's sense that he is in the process of ending life, when they consider admission, even if the patient or family cannot get a doctor to corroborate the sense that life is ending. It strikes me that it would not hurt the hospice movement if, once in a great while, someone who is not dying enters the hospice, makes his peace with the process of dying, and then gets well. It does seem to me profoundly damaging that people who are dying, but cannot document it, may never be admitted to a hospice and will not receive hospice care.

R H   What's the worst experience that you have had as a hospice volunteer?

J K   I haven't been active long enough to say that there was anything that was "worst." There are moments of awful grief, but all of them very rich — in the sense of human beings together, even in sadness. It's terrible to see someone in pain. There does come a time, I suppose, when you can't medicate someone without killing them outright. But there has to be a way to make someone comfortable. You want to do something, anything — hold them, rub them, roll them over.

The deterioration of the body in the last stages of illness is awful. It's always a shock to see someone who is not much more than a skeleton, albeit a skeleton who moves. I remember what it was like when my own body wasn't working. I felt this terrible alienation of me from my body a lot of the time. There was this really terrific energetic human being trapped in this rotten, broken body. Maybe this sense of separation of self from body makes me understand that the ravaged body is not the person. It's his body doing things that he doesn't have anything to say about.

I also wish that we had more opportunity to interact with the dying persons themeslves. Most of the patients who became part of our hospice don't do so until they are so far gone that there's almost nothing to do for them. The entire offering, then, is to the family. Of course, that's obviously worth a great deal.

I wish there was more time to do for the patient while the patient's "self" is still there. By the time a lot of patients come to the hospice, that patient's self is really gone. The patient is unconscious or very close to it and there isn't anything left but a body that is sort of working out its last energies. My sense is that it takes a family a long time to accept the prognosis of death, and often so long that they don't come to the point of being able to ask for help in the process of dying until it's just undeniable.

I am sorry at this point that I can't find out more about whether my own sense of dying can be corroborated by people who are, in fact, dying — or believe themselves to be or are believed to be. I'm sorry that I don't have the chance to share that information and build on it.

R H   Do you think the hospice movement will grow, will pick up momentum?

J K   I certainly hope so. I think so. We've spent a long, long time ignoring the end of life. I suppose for a long time we could because people didn't have a long time to die in most cases. One sickened and died. The process was short, often not very sweet, but pretty short.

I think the hospice movement has to grow because medi-

cal technology is available to prolong the process of living
and of dying. The implications of this are going to be felt
further and further in all directions and well into the future.
People who by all rights ought not to be alive will be alive,
in various states, for a long time. And they will need people
who care about them.

Part III
THE DILEMMA

I N other sections of this book, persons intimately involved in hospice care have discussed this concept from many perspectives. To a person, they are convinced that hospice represents a viable and needed alternative to the traditional care given to terminally ill patients, that it represents a better way to die. The need for this better way to die will be underscored by the population change that is taking place in this country — a change that may well test the viability of the concept.

Conservatively estimated, there will be more than 41 million people in this country over the age of 60 in the year 2000.[1] In that same year — barring miracle cures — 500,000 people are expected to die of cancer. Some of these more than 41 million people will have other terminal illnesses, some will have chronic diseases. Many of these persons will not need and, in many cases, will not want institutional care.

Where and how, then, will we care for those persons for whom recovery is no longer possible? In the last twenty years, the number of hospitals and total number of hospital beds have remained relatively stable, increasing and decreasing slightly over the years. In 1960, there were 6876 hospitals, having a total of 1,658,000 beds. In 1980, there were more hospitals, but fewer beds — 6965 hospitals and 1,365,000 beds.[2]

---

[1] Illustrative Projections of World Population to the 21st Century, Current Population Reports, Series P23, No. 79, 1979.
[2] Hospitals listed by the American Hospital Association in *Hospital Statistics*, 1961 and 1981 editions.

Statistics published in 1977, the latest statistics available, show there were 18,900 nursing homes, with 1,402,400 beds, in the reporting period covered.[3] Will traditional patterns of care be able to adjust to the changing, aging population and accommodate the kind of care needed? Can or should palliative care, as reflected in the hospice concept, fit into the current delivery system? If it can, where will palliative care fit? If it can't fit into the system and into the existing funding mechanisms, how will it be financed?

---

[3] National Health Statistics, Series 13, No. 43 (Washington, D.C.: G.P.O., 1977).

Chapter 14

WHERE DOES IT FIT?

THE health care delivery system in the United States is probably one of the most complex, and sometimes most unfathomable, in the western world. To understand where the hospice can or might fit into the existing system, it might be helpful to understand the organization of the system.

Institutional care in this country is, basically, provided by hospitals, long-term care institutions (more commonly known as nursing homes and convalescent homes), and rehabilitation institutions. In 1980, 6965 hospitals, with a total of 1,365,000 beds, were listed by the American Hospital Association in its *Guide Issue*, probably the most accurate count of inpatient institutions available. More than 60 percent of these hospitals have fewer than 100 beds. In 1977, the latest statistics available from the Center for Health Statistics, indicated there were 18,900 nursing homes with a total of 1,402,400 beds.

The American Hospital Association classifies hospitals by length of stay (short-term and long-term), by the major type of service (e.g., psychiatric), and by control, which represents the organizational control — government (federal, state, local), investor-owned (for profit), and community (not-for-profit).

Short-term or acute-care hospitals provide a variety of services depending, for example, on the size of the institution, the demand for services, competing providers, financial resources, target population, etc. A large, sophisticated urban hospital may offer not only acute-care inpatient services, but also outpatient or ambulatory care services in outpatient clinics, such as ear, nose, and throat clinics, and home care programs for persons who

161

need health care services but not hospitalization. Many of these same hospitals provide health education and community outreach programs, such as hypertension clinics. Some have smoking clinics, child abuse and neglect programs, drug abuse programs, and other types of support programs, such as crisis intervention "hotlines." Some of them also incorporate extended care or long-term care facilities in an effort to provide a continuum of care for their patients.

In all probability, services, programs, and therapies provided by these institutions include neurology service, nuclear medicine services, psychiatric services, coronary care units, burn units, intensive care units, neonatal intensive care units, radiation therapy, chemotherapy, cobalt therapy, and physical and occupational therapy. Most of these are, or represent, high-technology, curative services.

Smaller and less sophisticated hospitals — usually in small towns or rural areas — often provide only basic medical and surgical services. More sophisticated services are not available for a number of reasons. Among them are lack of specialized professional manpower, lack of community resources to support the costly equipment and the highly paid professionals needed to provide the services, and lack of enough demand to make the program or service viable.

Nursing homes also provide different types of services. In general, there are three levels of nursing care, and any given nursing home may provide one or all three of them. These levels of care — sheltered care, intermediate care, and skilled nursing care — are based on the physical and medical needs of the patient. Sheltered care patients are those who need the least care. They need, mainly, supervision of medication and nutrition and some help with personal care. Intermediate care patients require medical supervision and some nursing care, much of which can be provided by licensed practical nurses and nursing aides. Skilled nursing care patients require medical supervision and the highest level of nursing care, most of which is provided by registered nurses.

Health care services are provided by other, noninstitutional organizations, such as freestanding outpatient clinics; surgicenters, which provide surgical procedures on an outpatient basis; the new, nonhospital emergency centers; home health agencies; and health maintenance organizations, which focus first on preventive care and then on curative care. Where and how does hospice fit into this complex and fragmented system? — almost anywhere and everywhere and sometimes uncomfortably so. As shown in the diagram on the following page, almost every segment of the delivery system is providing hospice care — inpatient and/or home care. Community groups are also developing independent hospice programs, usually with hospital affiliation or back-up. Sometimes the back-up is simply by virtue of the medical director's or a team physician's medical privileges in one or more hospitals. Home health agencies and other community-based groups are also providing hospice care. Nursing homes are beginning to add hospice units or wings.

A large urban hospital may have an inpatient unit or wing, a hospice team that cares for terminally ill patients throughout the institution, and/or a team that provides hospice services to patients in their homes. A very small percentage of hospice care is provided as inpatient hospital care.

There are inherent problems in providing inpatient hospice care in acute-care institutions, because the philosophies underlying the two kinds of care are diametrically opposed. The goals of today's acute-care hospital is sophisticated curative care and maintenance of life; the goal of the hospice is good palliative care and maintenance of dignity.

Hospice units and programs are organized and staffed differently than medical/surgical units in the average hospital. They are usually governed by different policies and procedures.

If a hospital has a hospice unit, instead of a program providing care to the terminally ill patients throughout the hospital, that unit is likely to look considerably different from the other units. Efforts are usually made to make the environment as homelike as possible, to make it as un-institutional as possible. Nurses usually wear street clothes or modern colored uniforms instead of starched white uniforms and caps. Often there are lounges and kitchens and overnight accommodations, to provide meeting places and support services for the patient and members of his family. At Illinois Masonic Medical Center, for example, the small inpatient

HOSPICE: FITTING INTO THE SYSTEM?

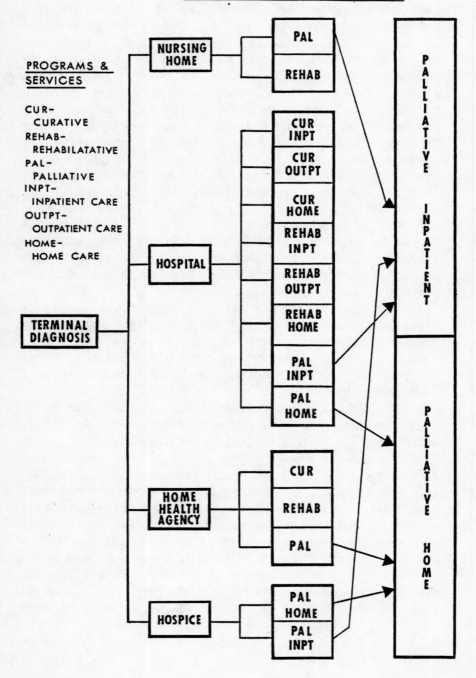

unit has a lounge and a small kitchenette, where family members may brew coffee or fix favorite foods for the patient. Families are also encouraged to eat meals with loved ones.

Hospice care is, by definition, provided by a multi-disciplinary team working closely together, with overall supervision provided by a physician. While team care is to be hoped for throughout the hospital, care is usually provided on the basis of the "captain of the ship" theory, with the physician being the undisputed captain who is in control at all times.

Because of the "hands-on" nature of hospice care, there is usually a higher staff/volunteer to patient ratio, with more care being given by volunteers than in other parts of the hospital. (It is interesting to note, however, that inpatient hospice programs provide more intensive medical and nursing care and use fewer volunteers than home care programs do.) Families are also encouraged to help with the actual physical care of the patient and are not asked to step out of the room when there is some nursing procedure to be done.

The pace in the hospice unit is slower than in other units because there is no rigid routine of tests and checks. The most important routine is that of providing medication on schedule – a schedule that keeps the pain cycle from beginning.

Because of such different philosophies of care, there are usually different policies and procedures governing hospice units or programs. The patient and the family is the unit of care. The goal is to make it possible for them to be together as much as possible, to share the last few precious moments together. Relaxing the visiting hours and rules is one way of doing this. Relaxing of rules can cause problems in an acute-care hospital. Even in institutions with long visiting hours, the visiting hours are not unlimited. In addition, most hospitals have rules preventing visits by children under a certain age. At Illinois Masonic Medical Center's Barr Pavillion, children of all ages are welcome. If it weren't for Board of Health regulations, there are some who would like to welcome the family pet.

It remains to be seen just how well two different philosophies and two different goals and two different rules and regulations can exist under one roof, or at least one organizational structure –

with one representing the existing health care model and the other, the new kid on the block, trying to find its niche. The hospice unit or wing appears better able to coexist with acute-care medicine than a program that provides hospice care to terminally ill patients wherever they are located in the hospital. The overlapping lines of authority are not nearly so discrete.

Organizationally, hospice care may, perhaps, be more comfortably located in a nursing home, where goals relate to rehabilitation or custodial care rather than cure. However, it is open to question whether the average nursing home is able to or will want to consistently provide a multi-disciplinary team of caregivers and enough volunteers to meet the goals of good hospice care. If the nursing home is investor-owned, the care may be too costly. If the nusing home is government-owned, the program will be competing for scarce resources with every other program.

Freestanding hospice institutions have been the goal of many fledgling hospice programs — a goal that does not seem practical in today's economy and in today's system. Instead of having freestanding hospices along the lines of the British model, some hospices are trying affiliations with other health care facilities to provide space for hospice patients to stay for a few days so that family members will have a brief respite from the toll-taking care they are giving to a loved one or a place for the patient to die, if the family can no longer deal with the prospect of having its loved one die at home.

Community-based, all volunteer programs that do not have to fit into an organizational structure provide, perhaps, the purest form of hospice care. Their survival is in question because of the need to continue to be in the fund-raising business. Even if all workers are volunteers and unpaid, it takes funding to maintain and operate the program, and it takes money to make money.

The question still remains, where does the hospice fit into the existing system?

What appears to be needed is a restructuring of the health care system, on the basis of epidemiology, in which the focus of care is on the type of care provided, not on the institutions or facility in which care is given. Such a restructuring would provide a single continuum of care, from preventive to curative to rehabilitative to palliative care. It would be a continuum through which the patient goes normally and naturally. The patient or family would not have to search out their options, then make value judgements that they may not be equipped to do knowledgeably or emotionally. This continuum would have further implications for our health care delivery system. It would have a great impact, for example, on medical and nursing education programs, which would have to incorporate training in palliative care.

When and if all doctors and nurses understand and use techniques of palliative care, the hospice per se will be obsolete.

Chapter 15

IS IT VIABLE FINANCIALLY?

FINANCING health care will be a major concern as we move toward the twenty-first century — for the providers of care, for patients, potential patients, and their families, for the federal government, and for providers of health care insurance.

It will be a major concern for the government, because the over-sixty population is increasing and the tax-base population is shrinking, which will result in even more competition for the tax dollar. Nongovernmental providers of insurance will also be affected by the changes in the population and the changes in the economy.

Given the aging population in this country, there will be an increase in the numbers of people who will develop chronic and terminal illnesses. Given the wonders of advanced technology, these people will be living longer. By the year 2000 hospitals and nursing homes will be hard pressed to care for the elderly ill, in terms of both beds and staff. These trends will bring with them social problems and health care delivery problems.

Ironically, the great advances in medical technology now require us to find viable alternatives, philosophically and financially, to some well-entrenched patterns of care.

Hospice is an alternative form of care that addresses both concerns. The first two parts of this book give testimony to the validity of the philosophical alternative of dying in one's own time and in one's own way, of dying pain free, surrounded by love and affection. Many hospice patients die at home. Others are cared for at home throughout most of the terminal stage of the illness, but go into the hospital for the last day or days.

It is the home care thrust of hospice that also speaks to the economics of health care. It has been estimated that home care hospice costs are about half of hospital costs. The difference will vary from program to program and from institution to institution. Even so, hospice care in general, and home hospice care in particular, have been proved to be less costly than inpatient care in an acute-care hospital.

Until hospice care made it possible for more terminally ill persons to be cared for at home, the hospital and the nursing home were the only options available to the patient and his family. Persons in the terminal stages of cancer for example (which represent 90% of all hospice patients) were taken to the acute-care hospital. In the hospital, they were kept alive as long as medical science could keep them alive, because that is the orientation of acute-care medicine. As a result, the already high cost of inpatient care was made even higher by the prolongation of life, regardless of the quality of the life that was being prolonged.

Consider simply the cost of being in a bed in an acute-care hospital. The cost can range from under $100 a day in a small rural hospital to more than $400 a day in an urban medical center. For this basic amount, the patient receives "bed and board" and around-the-clock nursing care. Add to this the cost of sophisticated, routine tests and procedures, e.g. checking the electrolyte balance every five hours, and the cost of high-technology monitoring equipment or any other sophisticated equipment should they be needed. Also add to the basic rate the cost of any other ancillary services that might be given to the patient.

Now, compare these costs with the basic costs of providing hospice home care, costs that are allocated much differently even though the services are available twenty-four hours a day. The major costs in most home care programs are the cost of medication and the cost of any skilled nursing services needed. Sometimes the costs include the services of such health care personnel as home health aides and licensed practical nurses. Usually, however, most of the physical care that would be provided in the hospital by a registered nurse or a licensed practical nurse is provided in the home by family members or volunteers.

In many, if not most, home care programs, only the nurses and volunteers visit the home on a regular basis. Most other members of the team — social workers, pastoral counselors, and nutritionists — come as requested or needed. Depending on the type and the stage of the illness, the nurse may visit once a week or maybe two or three times a week. Skilled nursing care is often needed more frequently at the end of the illness. It is conceivable that, in any given week, the hospice patient might be visited once by a physical therapist, and the patient and the patient's family might be visited once or twice by a social worker and a pastoral counselor. In the same week, the patient might be visited by the physician member of the team.

The frequency of visits by each of these team members will depend not only on the stage of the illness, but also on the physical, spiritual, emotional, and psychological needs of the members of the family.

For the sake of a cost comparison, the cost of basic components of care (bed and board and nursing care) in one Chicago hospital is $319 per day, minimum, for a two-bed room. In Chicago, the basic rate for a home visit by a registered nurse is $50 − 55. Should a home health aide be needed that day, add another $15 − 20. This totals less than $100 for that day, even if some estimate can be made for the cost of "bed and board" at home. What's more, in most cases, the patient does not need the nurse to visit every day.

As in a hospital, visits from other professionals — if the hospice is not an all-volunteer program — will add to the cost, as with medications needed. Often, however, medication is more expensive in the hospital than in the local pharmacy.

Today, the provision of health care is basically divided into preventive, curative, rehabilitative, and palliative care. As shown in the diagram in Chapter 14, these types of care can and are being given in different settings and configurations. This complicates the delivery of care and reimbursement for it.

In the past, commercial insurance companies and Medicare covered curative care and rehabilitative care, but not palliative care. Given the trend of an aging population, with the potential for life-threatening illnesses, caring for the terminally ill becomes a social problem as well as a health care delivery problem.

The recently successful effort to amend Medicare legislation to cover hospice care will bring with it the need to develop uniform standards of care and criteria for what constitutes hospice care for the purpose of state licensure. Standards and guidelines will also have to be developed as the basis of eligibility for reimbusement when it comes.

Until total palliative care — including the psychosocial elements — becomes an integral and reimbursable part of the delivery system, some arrangement will have to be made for covering the cost of palliative care, wherever that care is given. Bringing palliative care into the mainstream of medical care and making it an integral part of the continuum will require basic changes in medical education and, perhaps, a generation or two of practitioners.

EPILOGUE

BECAUSE it comes to each of us, death represents the natural end of life. But if it is to be accepted for what it is, we in America must come to a new understanding and acceptance of the dying person — of his needs, his fears, his concerns.

Earlier in this book, Jean Knoll poignantly expressed the loneliness and isolation of the person who is dying — or believes he is dying. Cindy Mitchell spoke with sadness and bewilderment about her mother's abandonment by her physician during the last days of her life. Dr. Sage talked wistfully about words left unsaid because a patient "died too soon," while Dr. Feldman talked about the needs of the dying patient and the ideal setting for his care. Kathy Woods spoke quietly about maximizing hope, and Randy Hughes marveled at the care given his sister by a hospice in California.

Only when the dying person is truly accepted again in society will the health care system be reshaped into whatever structure will best accommodate a true continuum of care — preventative, curative, rehabilitative, and palliative care. Just as death is an integral part of the life cycle, so caring for the dying person — in a manner consistent with his needs and wishes — should be an integral part of our health care system.

SELECTED BIBLIOGRAPHY*

Bhaduri, Reba. Care of the terminal patient — a family's sorrow. *Nursing Times 75:* 638 April 12, 1979.

Breitung, Joan. Attitudes toward the dying patient. *Nursing Care* 8:34 June 1975.

Breuer, Judith. Sharing a tragedy. *American Journal of Nursing* 76:758 May 1976.

Brinigion, Jeanne. Living with dying. *Nursing 78* 8(9):76 September 1978.

Central Office of Information, London. From the Reference Division: *Hospice Care in Britain*, March 1978.

Choron, Jacques. *Death and Western Thought*. New York: Colliers Books, 1963.

Cope, Lewis. To let people live until they die. *Minneapolis Tribune*, July 16, 1978.

Cowper-Smith, Frances. On the spot: mending the broken spirit. *Nursing Times* 75:772 May 10, 1979.

Craven, J. and Wald, F.S. Hospice care for dying patients. *American Journal of Nursing* 75:1816 October 1975.

Dempsey, David. *The Way We Die*. New York: Macmillan Co., 1975

Dobihal, E.F. Jr. Talk or terminal care? *Connecticut Medicine* 38:364 July 1974.

Dorang, Edith S. VNA — organized hospice volunteer program. *Nursing Outlook*, March 1981.

DuBois, Paul M. *The Hospice Way of Death*. New York: Human Sciences Press, 1980.

Dumont, Richard G. and Foss, Dennis C. *The American View of Death: Acceptance or Denial?* Cambridge, Mass.:Schenkman Publishing Company, Inc, 1972.

Experts probe issues around hospice care. *Hospitals* 54(10):63 June 1, 1980.

Feifel, Herman, ed. *Death in Contemporary America: New Meanings of Death*. New York: McGraw-Hill, Inc., 1977.

---

*A comprehensive bibliography is available from the National Hospice Organization, 1311A Dolley Madison Boulevard, McLean, Virginia 22101

────. *The Meaning of Death.* New York: McGraw-Hill, Inc., 1959.

Garfield, Charles, ed. *Psychosocial Care of the Dying Patient.* San Francisco: School of Medicine, University of California, 1976.

Hamilton, M. and Reid, H.A., eds. *Hospice Handbook.* Grand Rapids, Mich.: Wm. B. Eerdmans, 1980.

Holden, Constance. The hospice movement and its implications. *ANNALS* 447:59 January 1980.

Ingles, Thelma. St. Christopher's Hospice. *Nursing Outlook* 22:759 December 1974.

International Work Group in Death, Dying, and Bereavement. Assumptions and principles underlying standards for terminal care. *American Journal of Nursing* 79:297.

Kastenbaum, R. Towards standards of care for the terminally ill: a few guiding principles. *Omega* 7:191.

Kastenbaum, R. and Aisenberg, R. *The Psychology of Death.* New York: Springer Publishing Company, 1972.

Kohn, J. Hospice movement provides humane alternative for terminally ill patients. *Modern Health Care* 6:26 September 1976.

Kolbe, Richard. The English hospice. *Hospitals* 51:65.

Kubler-Ross, Elisabeth. *Living with Death and Dying.* New York: Macmillan, Inc., 1981.

────. *On Death and Dying.* New York: Macmillan, Inc., 1969.

────. *Questions and Answers on Death and Dying.* Macmillan, Inc., 1974.

Lamerton, R.C. The need for hospices. *Nursing Times* 71:155 January 23, 1975.

Martin, Ann. Hospice nursing. *Nursing 81* 11(2):128 February 1981.

McNairn, Noreen. Helping the patient who wants to die at home. *Nursing 81* 11(2):66 February 1981.

Pattison, E. *The Experience of Dying.* Englewood Cliffs, N.J.: Prentice-Hall, Inc., 1977.

Plant, Janet. Finding a home for hospice care in the United States. *Hospitals* 51:53 July 1, 1977.

Quint, J.C. *The Nurse and the Dying Patient.* New York: Macmillan, Inc., 1967.

Saunders, Cicely. And from sudden death. *Nursing Times* 58:1045 August 17, 1962.

────. Hospice care. *Journal of the American Medical Association* 65:726 1979.

────, ed. *The Management of Terminal Diseases.* London: Edward Arnold, Ltd., 1978.

Schoenberg, B., et al. *Anticipatory Grief.* New York: Columbia University Press, 1974.

────. *Loss and Grief: Psychological Management in Medical Practice.* New York: Columbia University Press, 1970.

Shubin, Seymour, ed. How to work more comfortably with grief: your own and your patient's. *Nursing Life* 1(1):55 July/August 1981.

Silver, Susan. A way to prolong living, rather than dying. *Chicago Tribune,* November 7, 1978.

Sister Paula. Care of the terminally ill — the work of the hospice. *Nursing Times* 75:667 April 19, 1979.

Stoddard, Sandol. *The Hospice Movement.* Briarcliff Manor, N.Y.: Stein and Day Publishers, 1980.

Ufema, Joy. Do you have what it takes to be a nurse-thanatologist? *Nursing* 77 7(5):96 May 1977.

U.S. Public Health Service and American Nursing Foundation. *An Interdisciplinary Study of Care of Dying Patients and their Families.* F.W. Wald, Principal Investigator (USPHS Grant No. NU 00325-06, Grant 2-70-023).

Wald, Florence S., Foster, Zelda, and Wald, Henry J. The hospice movement as a health care reform. *Nursing Outlook* 28(3):173 March 1980.

Ward, Barbara J. Hospice home care program. *Nursing Outlook* 26(10):646 October 1978.

Zorza, Victor and Zorza, Rosemary. *A Way to Die.* New York: Knopf, 1980.

INDEX

179